The FOUR FORCES of Human Nature

A Unifying Theory

Roberto Treviño Peña

Illustrations by Marie Ferrante

Fulton Books
Meadville, PA

Published by Fulton Books 2024

ISBN 979-8-88982-371-1 (paperback)
ISBN 979-8-89221-989-1 (hardcover)
ISBN 979-8-88982-372-8 (digital)

Printed in the United States of America

To my wife, Maria del Carmen, who was my anchor
as I tethered out into space and dwelled into the cells
to understand the workings of human nature.

CONTENTS

Introduction

Since physicists discovered the four fundamental forces of nature—strong, weak, electromagnetic (EM), and gravity—they have tried to unify them into one theory. Physicists went down to the subatomic level to search and ended up with vibrating strings. They went up into space and ended up with gravitons (which are yet to be found). But what do these forces mean in terms of human behavior? In *The Four Forces of Human Nature: A Unifying Theory*, I connect the four fundamental forces of physics with the four forces of human nature. I identify the four human forces and the specific brain areas responsible for processing them. Then I explain how the interaction of these forces influences human behavior.

The four human forces are affective, cognitive, communicative, and socio-environmental. The aim of these is to get, keep, and increase the four human necessities: health, status, wealth, and basic drives (eat, sleep, sex). Every person needs the four necessities for self-preservation. Without these necessities, humans can die prematurely or become extinct as a species!

Different brain areas are responsible for processing each of the affective, cognitive, communicative, and socio-environmental forces. The processing centers for each of these are, respectively, the amygdala, thalamus, cerebral cortex, and insular cortex.

What is the analogy between the four fundamental forces of physics and the four forces of human nature? The strong, weak, EM, and gravity forces correspond, in the same order, to the affective, cognitive, communicative, and socio-environmental forces. The *strong force* is stronger than the *weak force*; humans are more passionate than they are rational. The *strong force* holds the nucleus together; the *affective force* objective is self-preservation. The *weak force* is involved in the change and transformation of particles; the *cognitive force* is involved in the change and transformation of individuals. The *EM force* is the interaction that occurs between particles and is mediated by photons and radio waves; the *communicative force* is the interaction that occurs between individuals, and it is mediated mostly by photons and sound waves. *Gravity* is an attractive force; it causes bodies to be attracted to each other. The *socio-environment* is an attractive force; it produces an affinity among humans and nature.

Furthermore, the weak and EM forces (electroweak) were the first to be unified into a single force; the cognitive and communicative forces are unified in the upper brain. There is an indication that the strong force unifies with the electroweak force at higher energies; the affective, cognitive, and communicative forces are unified within the human brain. EM and gravity forces are related. Both are associated with ripples in the fabric of space. The communicative and socio-environmental forces are related. Both are associated with communications back and forth within the fabric of space. As you read along the book you will understand better the analogy between physics and neuroscience.

The Power of Force

Force is a power that puts an object in motion and makes something happen. In this book, we are going to consider force specifically as it relates to humans—*us*. Humans' affective, cognitive, communicative, and socio-environmental forces are powerful—so powerful that they influence or move a person in a certain direction. Thus, force is a vector quantity; it has both a magnitude and direction.

Force is a method to transfer energy. Say a parent tells her child to do his homework. The child walks to his room, picks up his schoolbooks, and begins doing homework. Without there being any physical contact between parent and child, there was a transfer of energy between the two that caused a movement.

The energy transferred had enough magnitude to move the child in a certain direction. In this case, magnitude is the number of hours spent studying and vector is the direction of going from C to

A school grades. Magnitude and vector also measure misdeeds. The number of hours a hacker spends on the computer to gain unauthorized access to data.

Brain Power

It is important to note here that the brain is a complex organ, and a simple behavior such as the child walking to his room activates millions of neurons and many brain parts within the child. This is because no brain part operates in isolation. Although walking activates the left and right and upper and lower brain parts, there is one brain part that rules—the cerebellum. The cerebellum's predominant role is motor control. Similar to this book, many brain parts are involved in human behavior, but the "processing centers" predominate.

In this book, therefore, I will explain in detail the predominant roles of the amygdala, thalamus, cerebral cortex, and insular cortex in regard to the forces of human nature. I want you to know in advance, however, that this will be a bit of an oversimplification so as not to lose you, the reader, in the thick forest of brain circuitry.

With the advent of newer medical technology instruments, it is now a good time to study and understand the workings of the brain. Electrical diagnostic tools such as electrocorticography and electroencephalography record the electrical activity of the brain. Neuroimaging techniques such as magnetic resonance imaging (MRI) and positron emission tomography (PET) visualize the activity of brain parts while study participants perform certain tasks or just think. And brain surgery procedures, such as stereotaxic surgery with microelectrode recording and brain stimulations using electrical probes, demonstrate the effect of brain parts on certain body movements. While it is beyond the scope of this book to give detailed explanations as to how these diagnostic tools work, this book will elaborate on the workings of the brain using the findings from these diagnostic tools.

Research Behind the Findings

This book is based on theory and practice. *Theory* is what you know, and *practice* is applying what you know to real situations. It is based on your author Roberto Treviño Peña's extensive knowledge and experience conducting studies supported by the National Institutes of Health, the US Department of Agriculture, and the US Department of Health and Human Services. In his career, he has been the principal investigator of some of the largest clinical trials aimed at understanding and improving health behaviors and biological markers of disease in both children and adults. While many investigators spend their professional career finding the causes of disease, others spend it exploring solutions to mitigate disease. Dr. Treviño Peña chose to focus on the latter: exploring solutions to disease burdens. This book is therefore the outcome of his decades-long experience in medical and neuroscientific research. This book is aimed at both lay audiences and experts.

Many of the papers referenced in this book are from literature reviews and meta-analyses. *Literature review* is when scientists collect many of the best design studies from around the world to analyze and offer conclusive findings on a specific subject. *Meta-analysis* is a statistical method for combining and integrating the results of multiple studies on a given subject to come up with a quantitative summary. Meta-analyses are considered the highest level of evidence for scientific discoveries. When I was searching the general literature on the physiology of the amygdala, for example, I discovered hundreds of articles from around the world, and these did not include studies on animals. So I narrowed the literature search for this book mostly to articles on humans from around the world that were written as literature reviews or using meta-analysis.

Still, science is an evolving field, so what is conclusive today may not be conclusive tomorrow. You also should know that while the findings in the book are referenced with the most up-to-date articles, some of the books and published studies that I cite are those which have withstood the test of time. Examples are David Hume's

The Treatise of Human Nature (1738) and St. Thomas Aquinas's *Summa Theologica* (1274).

The Book's Scope

I have written this book so the reader—the *individual*—will start to reflect on the extremely powerful forces he or she possesses. Within this book, the terms *individual, necessities,* and *forces* are given special significance. This is because it is the individual who is in search of the four necessities and it is within the individual that the forces operate to get, keep, and increase the four necessities.

The focus of this book is *physiology* (the study of the functions and mechanisms of the brain) and not *pathophysiology* (neurological and psychiatric disorders). As a person begins to understand the functions of the brain and the influence that the socio-environment has on it, the methods to promote health become clearer and more achievable. I state health because it is my specialty, and if the individual has good health, he or she can more readily take on the task to get, keep, and increase the other three necessities.

CHAPTER 1

Affective Force
The First Responder

The affective force is a combination of activities in the body and mind that act as the link connecting your emotions to the world. This connection is electrifying. This electricity excites you or dulls you. It exuberates or depresses you.[1] In this way, the affective force creates our self-worth and meaning. The affective force is the soul of the body. It is this vital affective force that will be explored throughout the first chapter.

The purpose of the affective force is to defend against perceived threats. It does so by appraising incoming stimuli as appetitive or aversive.[2] In this book, favorable or rewarding events are referred to as *appetitive*, and unfavorable or punishing events are referred to as *aversive*. This appraisal by the affective force is intentional, meaning it is directed at a particular cause—the stimulus (which may or may not be real).[3] We will deal with this later in the chapter.

We become aware of physical responses when the affective force perceives an event as appetitive or aversive. For instance, the affective force can turn on the autonomic nervous system (shown through sweating or a rapid heart rate), incite a passion (perhaps one of anger or joy), and manifest a behavior (fight or flight). People welcome events that produce appetitive impressions and avoid events that produce aversive ones. However, research shows that aversive events make stronger impressions than appetitive events (by an estimated ratio of 2.5:1.5).[4] Therefore, aversive stimuli receive more attention than appetitive ones. This is why emotionally negative experiences may override the positive memories in your mind!

Real or Not?

Before describing the principles underlying the affective force, it is important to understand how incoming stimuli are perceived. Incoming stimuli can originate from outside of us or inside of us. *Exteroceptive* stimuli originate from the social environment; *interoceptive* stimuli come from within the person. A person receives exteroceptive stimuli through sensory organs (e.g., seeing or hearing), whereas interoceptive stimuli are prompted by self-reflections (via a person's imagination). For example, if a candidate for a particular position receives a letter stating he "got the job" it will produce an exteroceptive stimulus (from the environment). The affective force appraises the exteroceptive stimulus as appetitive because it is something to be desired. On the other hand, if that same person is lying in bed trying to go to sleep and, through self-reflection, retrieves embarrassing memories of his interview, this will produce an interoceptive stimulus that the affective force appraises as an aversive event (an internal stimulus that is undesirable).

It is important to note that the affective force often makes appraisals of exteroceptive and interoceptive stimuli based on imagination rather than on observation. Imagination can be illusory, and observation derives from facts. To clarify:

- *Imagination in the realm of fantasy* is when a person makes an appraisal based on a perception that is not real. On top of that, the appraisal may be tinged with preconceptions, such as biases, prejudices, predispositions, or inclinations. For example, a job candidate walks out of her interview feeling that she did not get the job (even though the interviewer gave no feedback). Perhaps this candidate has preconceived notions that the interview went awry because she is obese and has previously been shamed for her weight. Based on this preconception, the job seeker imagines (unjustifiably) that she will not be hired because the interviewer is biased against her weight.

- *Observation* is when a person makes an appraisal based on an existing fact. For example, the job seeker gets a letter in the mail with a job offer. The letter is the fact (i.e., observation) that the job interview went well.

Fortunately, preconceptions are not necessarily bad or harmful. In fact, preconceptions are important for everyday interactions because they create the platform on which we retain, abandon, or change our perspectives. Since many of the affective force's appraisals are based on illusion, let's take an even deeper look at the potential side effects of imagination. We'll use the previous example of the dejected job seeker.

In this example, the job seeker may be feeling sad due to her imagined bias of being judged adversely. Sadness may make her miserable, causing her to lose sleep and be irritable toward others. The unpleasant emotion (sadness) and behavior (lack of sleep) can be depressing—but even more harmful is the activation of the autonomic nervous system. In response to the affective force's appraisal, the nervous system produces stress hormones (corticosteroids and norepinephrine) that elevate blood pressure, increase blood sugars, and cause stomach ulcers. As you might guess, this is not a healthy condition for the body.

Consider this, though: All these unhealthy side effects were produced because of an appraisal that was faulty or unfounded at the time. The person didn't even know whether she got the job! In this example, the individual's imagination stops, and observation appears only once an official job offer or rejection occurs.

Consider another example of an imagination-based appraisal by the affective force. Let's say a worker walks into the workplace and walks past a colleague without greeting him. The colleague then begins to imagine that the coworker is upset at him. As a result of the faulty assumption, he may feel anger toward her, thinking, "Why was she so rude? I haven't done anything to her!" This series of events may cause him to start acting negatively toward the coworker.

The anger that the individual is experiencing now causes an increase is the secretion of stress hormones such as cortisol; these, in turn, will make him even more miserable (he recognizes he is tired, fatigued, and extremely irritable). Now remember, this whole experience was based on imagination rather than observation. Later in the day, the coworker informs her colleagues that her spouse was diagnosed with cancer and given only seven months to live. In this case, the individual had assumed the coworker personally disliked him (this was a figment of imagination) when in reality the coworker was upset because of her spouse's diagnosis which was the factual reality.

The affective force, which is a part of the primal brain, may mean well but can often drive people up a wall. The good news is that there is within us another force namely the cognitive force. This comes into play and gives the affective force some direction. Important appetitive or aversive events appraised by the affective force are transmitted to the cognitive force for further processing, storage, feedback, or action. Even so, the affective force is stronger than the cognitive force because it is (1) the first force activated when harm is present and (2) the first to press the emergency buttons and defend the individual. The interaction between the affective and cognitive forces will be further discussed in the next chapter.

The Principle of Self-Preservation Guided by Four Necessities

The appraisal process begs the question, "What principle does the affective force use to determine whether a stimulus is appetitive or aversive?" The answer is self-preservation. Self-preservation is indispensable for a person's well-being. In the absence of well-being, a person feels physical pain or mental anguish. The combination of these undesirable states can lead to premature death.

Therefore, self-preservation is a necessity. A necessity is different from a want (or wish) and a desire (or craving). Rather, a necessity is a need that a person must fulfill to survive. The four necessities that are important for a person's self-preservation are as follows:

1. Health
2. Status (interpersonal relationships)

3. Wealth
4. Basic drives (eating, sleeping, and having sex)

The affective force constantly appraises incoming stimuli to get, keep, and increase the four necessities. Not only are the four necessities important for a person's survival but they are also important to building the person's dignity and self-worth. It is important to note that increasing the four necessities does have its limits. As will be explained below, there is a fine balance between too little and too much of the four necessities.

An event that threatens the four necessities will engage the affective force with full power and strength. When threatened, the affective force acts spontaneously and out of our awareness; it does not even ask the cognitive force for permission! For example, the noise of a rattlesnake will make a person jump quickly away from the noise. Only later will the person consciously reflect on what the noise was, where it was located, and how to best avoid it. At that moment, the affective force acted swiftly to keep the person safe from the rattlesnake. Self-preservation and survival are the priority. Neurobiologically this is called the amygdala hijack. The amygdala takes over when the individual is under threat for an optimal response.

Shown below are brief examples of common threats to the four necessities. These are threats that will activate the affective force (see table 1). *Health* threats include events that could harm the body. For instance, a health threat could be something as simple as looking for oncoming cars before crossing the street. Health threats can also be more complex events, such as taking preventive measures against a heart attack by eating healthy and adopting an active lifestyle. *Status* threats can lead to a lack of connection or emotional pain in our relationships. Examples of status threats include social isolation, loneliness, and bullying. *Wealth* threats are threats to our financial well-being and access to resources. These threats could be as simple as lacking shelter for the night, or they could be more complex events, such as foreclosure on an expensive mansion. Last, threats to *basic drives* include anything that prevents us from engaging in the essential functions needed for survival. These threats involve a lack of eating, sleeping, and sex. (It is obvious that people need food and sleep to survive, and without sex, humanity would be extinct.)

Table 1. Human's four necessities	
Health	Status

1. Health promotion
2. Disease prevention
	1. Family
	   a. Immediate
	   b. Extended
	2. Friends
	   a. Intimate
	   b. Personal
	3. Peers
	   a. School
	   b. Work
	   c. Organizations
	4. Acquaintances

Wealth	Basic Drives
1. Money 2. Material items	1. Eat 2. Sleep 3. Sex

Note that *status* (as shown in table 1) means the position of a person in relation to another or others (i.e., a person's family, friends, and so on), and *wealth* means ownership of material items (clothing, car, mansion, and so on).

Why They Matter

The four necessities matter to each and every person to survive. The affective force, therefore, is a strong defender of these four necessities. When a person lacks just one necessity, the repercussions are enough to cause premature death. Systematic reviews from around the world have shown that some of the most common causes for suicide are failing health, loss of a partner (status), and financial stress (wealth).[5–7]

Since the four necessities are so important, a person may justify "going to the extreme" is necessary to ensure that these needs are met. You may be tempted to drop excessive amounts of body weight, work out constantly, have a large circle of friends, make wealth generation a priority, or sleep all the time. However, an excess of any of these can also cause physical pain or mental anguish. There is a fine balance that must be kept.

While each of the four necessities are important on their own each has an impact on self-preservation independent of one another and in addition, they also impact each other. Despite their independence, the necessities are not isolated points but four corners of the same square. They connect to each other, and what affects one affects all. For example, if a person's health worsens, it may affect their ability to maintain their wealth. If the person's wealth disappears, it may affect the status of their relationships in the family or with their landlord.

The lack of more than one necessity has a compounding effect. By this, I mean that the risk to someone's self-preservation doubles if a lack of one necessity leads to a lack of another necessity. The more the occurrence of lacks, the greater the risk.

Necessity 1
Health

According to the World Health Organization, health is a state of complete physical, mental, and social well-being. The absence of well-being implies the presence of physical pain or mental anguish. Therefore, the affective force is constantly attempting to prevent bodily injury and promote well-being. During the day, the force is "on guard" and ready to defend you against events that may cause physical pain and/or mental anguish.

Most of the time the affective force does its work at a subconscious level. For example, when you touch a hot stove, your body releases a subconscious motor reflex that removes your hand from the hot stove. Fractions of seconds later, that action becomes conscious, and you reflect on what happened during the event; this is delayed consciousness.[8] The pain avoidance act (i.e., removing your hand) was a subconscious reaction first and only a conscious act later on. Similarly, you might have had the experience of driving a car while your mind is occupied with work. However, while you are distracted you subconsciously choose to stop at stop signs and red lights. In this example, your affective force is a constant vigilante preserving your well-being, so you don't crash!

Moreover, the affective force is primitive in terms of its evolutionary origin, and it is also innate. Humans are born with basic defense mechanisms to prevent injury. Newborns have the grasp reflex (they hold on when falling), the startle reflex (they cover their body with their arms after a loud noise), and the unsettling cry (they cry to signal their need to eat, rest or relieve pain).[9] These reflexes are innate, subconscious, and facilitated by the affective force.

The concept of health is so essential that just believing you are in poor health can lead to bad health consequences over time. Scientists have developed self-rating health surveys that measure health problems, physical functioning, mental stress, and health behaviors.[10] Within these surveys, one question is where a person is asked, "How do you rate your health?" The responses offered are "poor," "fair," "good," "very good," or "excellent." Studies that use these surveys have shown the risk of dying from all causes significantly increased for those who perceived their health status as poor than those who perceived their health as excellent.[11, 12] So how a person perceives his or her health status appears to be a unique factor in determining their risk of death.

Everything in Moderation

Yet engaging in too much or too little of any necessity can prove unhealthy. A person who eats too much fatty food can suffer from a heart attack, but a person who eats too little fatty food (in a misguided attempt to prevent a heart attack) can end up suffering from a hormonal deficiency as fat is the core molecule needed to produce estrogen and testosterone. Similarly, taking a Tylenol can be good for a person's health or headache, but taking too much Tylenol can damage the liver. Moderation and balance are key when addressing the necessities!

In addition, the necessities are interconnected. Too much of one necessity can negatively affect another necessity! Let's pair the basic drives with health for a moment. A sedentary lifestyle and excessive eating can affect health in a negative way by causing obesity, and obesity is the common denominator of several chronic diseases.[13–16] In this example, your basic needs (activity, eating) affect your health (i.e., obesity, chronic disease). An excess or lack of one necessity will impact the other necessities.

Necessity 2
Status

The necessity of belonging is natural and instinctual. So saying "I don't care what other people think" might be an acceptable defense mechanism, but it is not deemed acceptable by the affective force!

The affective force is sensitive to social status as relationships with others (or the lack thereof) give humans validity—in other words, how family, friends, peers, or acquaintances view and value us means a lot.

The need to relate to others or to belong to a group is inherent in humans. Relationships are indispensable. We are social beings from birth! Within weeks of birth, newborns are more likely to cease crying when they hear their caregiver's voice versus the sound of a mechanical device.[17] Conversely, disruption of the mother-infant bond (due to rejection or abuse) has been associated with emotional and behavioral problems in childhood, such as hyperactivity, temper tantrums, and anxiety.[18, 19]

Status originates from our daily interactions and our more committed relationships.[17] Interactions are simple and usually of short duration; relationships are complex and usually long-lasting. A person forms interactions with acquaintances. A person forms relationships with family, friends, and peers. The exchanges that occur in both interactions and relationships are transactional. Verbal messages, exchange of goods, acts of service, and body language are all examples of transactions we have with other people.

Relationships require more engagement than interactions. The nature of connectedness and the quality of the time spent in a relationship are more important than that spent in the interactions. Relationships are driven by subcortical regions deep in the brain to satisfy a person's emotional well-being. Because of this subcortical nature, people can feel attraction or revulsion toward another person even without actually meeting them.

Not only is status important for our well-being, but social connection is essential for relieving stress. Humans are naturally inclined to reach out to others in stressful times. We seek other humans to relieve stress and maintain sanity.[20] In other words, people need other people to provide them with social support!

Such social support can be physical (health care), psychological (love, sympathy, empathy), or economic (jobs, tangible goods). Those who experience social support are more able to resist disease. If already suffering from a disease, those with social support have lower rates of hospitalization and recuperate faster.[17] In many ways, relationships are essential to our very survival.

Relate or Die Early

The effects of status, or lack thereof, have been studied extensively in humans. Scientists have assessed status by two types of instruments: those that measure social isolation[21] and those that measure loneliness.[22] Social isolation and loneliness are two constructs that measure different aspects of status. The instrument that measures social isolation is objective. Instruments that measure social isolation evaluate the frequency of the transactions. For instance, a survey assessing social isolation may ask, "Does the individual engage or interact with a spouse, parent, friend, or neighbor at least once every two weeks?" The response scales range from 1 (never) to 4 (very often).

Measuring loneliness elicits subjective responses. This instrument measures the feeling of being unhappy with one's relationships.

The test may ask, "How often do you feel alone? How often do you feel part of a group of friends? How often do you feel that you lack companionship? How often do you feel left out?" The response scales range from 1 (never) to 4 (very often).

Meta-analysis is a quantitative, formal, epidemiological study design used to systematically assess previous research studies to derive conclusions about that body of research., One such meta-analysis found that persons who reported being socially isolated and lonely had an increased likelihood of premature death (by 29 percent and 26 percent, respectively), as compared to those who reported a strong social network of support.[23]

A second meta-analysis reviewed two sets of studies: ones that used social isolation surveys and others that used loneliness surveys. The researchers wanted to determine the relationship between social isolation, loneliness, and cardiovascular disease. When the investigators combined the two sets of studies, results showed that participants with high levels of social isolation and loneliness had a 50 percent increased risk of cardiovascular disease.[24] A third meta-analysis also showed strong evidence that both social isolation and loneliness were associated with increased mortality, decreased mental health, low physical activity, and overeating.[25] Although both isolation and loneliness had undesirable effects, social isolation most consistently led to negative effects. The Beatles wrote best about the sadness of loneliness:

Eleanor Rigby

Ah, look at all the lonely people
Ah, look at all the lonely people

Eleanor Rigby
Picks up the rice in the church where a wedding has been
Lives in a dream
Waits at the window
Wearing the face that she keeps in a jar by the door
Who is it for?

All the lonely people
Where do they all come from?
All the lonely people
Where do they all belong?

Father McKenzie
Writing the words of a sermon that no one will hear
No one comes near
Look at him working
Darning his socks in the night when there's nobody there
What does he care?

All the lonely people
Where do they all come from?
All the lonely people
Where do they all belong?

Ah, look at all the lonely people
Ah, look at all the lonely people

Eleanor Rigby
Died in the church and was buried along with her name
Nobody came
Father McKenzie
Wiping the dirt from his hands as he walks from the grave
No one was saved

All the lonely people (ah, look at all the lonely people)
Where do they all come from?
All the lonely people (ah, look at all the lonely people)
Where do they all belong?

It is important to note that many factors can lead to stress and early death. Individuals experiencing low social support (status) may also be individuals with low economical resources (wealth). An argument could be made that lack of wealth, instead of lack of status, causes the stress reported by study participants. Indeed, a study of individuals who suffered a heart attack reported that both low social support and low economical resources were related to stress and death.[26] However, after the investigators controlled for level of income, individuals with low social support still had high rates of stress and death. This study concluded that status and wealth, independently of each other, are associated with poor mental and physical health outcomes.

Everything in Moderation

Too much status (i.e., too many relationships and interactions) also proves harmful. How can this be? One example is celebrities who are constantly followed and sought after. This is too much status. The lives of these celebrities have become overwhelmed by so much social interaction that they hardly have a private life anymore! Just ask Meghan Markle, who is married to Prince Harry. She has spoken openly about the mental health struggles that accompany fame. Because of their lack of personal space and privacy, many of these famous individuals may live frustrated, miserable lives. Some even take up drug addictions or commit suicide.

Necessity 3
Wealth

The drive to get, keep, and increase wealth is an inherent human necessity. Because the lack or loss of wealth is perceived as harmful to a person, the affective force acts as the first defense mechanism to protect and boost someone's wealth.

Wealth, in this book, is not defined as limited to an abundance of money and material resources. It includes any money and material items needed to keep the individual alive, such as having a dollar or two to buy a meal or the means to buy a coat to protect against freezing temperatures. In other words, wealth does not mean you are the richest person alive but that you have the material means to live.

Table 2. Methods used to measure wealth
• Educational attainment
• Household income
• Income inequality (Gini Coefficient)
• Poverty level (income plus number of people living in a household)
• Neighborhood deprivation (US census)
• Occupation
• Net worth (assets minus liabilities)
• Composite score of the above

Social scientists have studied the effects of wealth on individual well-being. There are many ways of measuring wealth, and there is no consensus as to which method is preferable (see table 2). Regardless of the method, the findings are the same: threats to wealth are harmful to humans. Thus, it is a necessity for the affective force to constantly appraise if the possession of wealth is being threatened, and to take measures to protect wealth from adversities.

On the low end of wealth is poverty. Poverty has been shown to have a causal relationship with disease. Studies have shown that poor people, when compared to their more affluent counterparts, have higher rates of stress, heart disease, diabetes, obesity, hypertension, and psychiatric illnesses. Financially disadvantaged people are also more susceptible to various cancers.[27–32]

Lack or loss of wealth is not just associated with disease. It is also related to death and life expectancy. A large study that measured neighborhood deprivation showed an excess of mortality among persons in "deprived" neighborhoods compared to those in affluent neighborhoods.[33] In men, living in the deprived neighborhoods had a 41 percent higher mortality rate than those living in the affluent neighborhoods. In women, the mortality rate was 77 percent higher in deprived neighborhoods compared to those living in affluent ones. Other studies have also found a strong relationship between poverty and early death.[29, 34–37]

On the opposite end of death is life expectancy—how long a person is expected to live. Sure enough, studies have found that people with more wealth live longer than those who have less wealth. One large study highlights this point. The study included 1.4 billion records, including income data obtained from de-identified tax records and mortality data from Social Security Administration death records.[38] In this study, the gap in life expectancy between the richest 1 percent and poorest 1 percent was 14.6 years for men and 10.1 years for women. The investigators also found that the higher the income, the higher the life expectancy throughout the income distribution.

The relationship between good health and income follows a linear gradient: the greater the wealth, the better the health.[39] Poverty affects health outcomes at every level without a cutoff. Others have also reported a gap in life expectancy between those with the most and those with the least wealth.[28, 36, 40–42]

What happens when there is a sudden change in one's financial circumstances—for example, when one is used to being wealthy and then suddenly suffers an economic downturn? Studies show that individuals who have a sudden loss of wealth have an increased rate of disease and early death. A sudden loss of net worth (homestead, business, retirement accounts, bank accounts, investments, vehicles) is known as *wealth shock*. A team of investigators first assessed for wealth shock in 1994 and continued conducting interviews biennially through 2014 (for twenty years).[43] *Wealth shock* was defined as a loss of 75 percent or more of total net worth over a two-year period. The wealth shock group studied had a median decrease in net worth of $101,568. This wealth shock group was compared with those who were in "asset poverty" (owed the same or more than what they owned) and those who did not have a wealth shock (median net worth increase of $13,894, a group known as the *reference group*).

When compared to the reference group, the mortality rate was 50 percent higher in the wealth shock group and 67 percent higher in the asset poverty group over the twenty-year period. Other investigators also found a significant relationship between wealth shock, disease, and premature death.[44–46]

These studies lead us to ask: Why does the lack or loss of wealth cause disease and premature death? It could be that lack or loss of wealth is not the direct cause of death. Scientists study causality by measuring mediators and moderators. (A *mediator* is the middleman, and a *moderator* is the third party.) It may be that the lack of wealth is mediated by a "middleman," such as a lack of health insurance coverage. So in this example, a lack of health insurance, not a lack of wealth, would be the direct cause of death.

Lack or loss of wealth → Lack of health insurance → Death

It is also possible that a moderator impacts the connection between wealth and premature death. A moderator weakens or strengthens the relationship between two variables. In this case, we are talking about the relationship between lack or loss of wealth and disease or premature death. For example, age could be a moderator between wealth and death. If this is the case, the relationship between wealth and death could be stronger for older people and less strong for younger people. In other words, older people may be more likely to experience premature death from lack or loss of wealth than younger people.

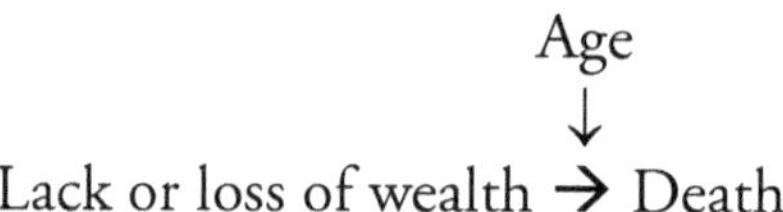

Furthermore, it is well known that poor people are more likely to be uninsured, lack access to medical care, receive substandard medical care, and belong to a minority ethnic group (who have higher rates of chronic disease and lower survival rates for disease). Each one of these factors could be a mediator or moderator that impacts the relationship between a person's wealth and health! But here is what is important to know: The studies used in this book controlled for mediators and moderators. This means that the researchers were able to analyze the relationship between wealth and early death on their own and without the impact of mediators or moderators. Because of this, we can know that lack or loss of wealth on its own is a direct cause of disease and death.

Status is a variable that can be associated with wealth. A national US study evaluated the interaction between status, wealth, and health with a survey of 16,044 participants.[47] It showed that the combination of social isolation and poverty on death was larger than isolation and poverty factors as individual contributors. This confirms that the four necessities are independent of each other. Taking all of this research together, we can know that lack of wealth on its own impacts a person's well-being.

Exactly How Does Poverty Cause Disease and Premature Death?

Now we know lack of wealth is responsible for causing disease and premature death. We must ask: By what mechanism does poverty cause disease or premature death?

Table 3. How the lack or loss of wealth can cause death	
Material Mechanisms	Psychological Mechanisms
• Inability to attain a higher level of education • Lack of health insurance • Suboptimal medical care • Lack of available transportation • Living in neighborhoods with food deserts • Living in neighborhoods predisposes to occupational hazards • Inferior housing • Discrimination	• Stress • Depression • Distrust • Feeling disrespect • Hopelessness • Feeling lonely

There are two trains of thought as to what is responsible for the relationship between wealth and health: material mechanisms and psychological mechanisms (see table 3).[48] The material mechanisms were discussed in the studies referenced above. The findings were that actual wealth, or material resources, were the direct cause of death.

The other mechanism is psychological—that it is the person's emotional and psychological state of mind that determines health outcomes. There is a strong indication that the psychological mechanism is the most powerful force affecting health outcomes. For instance, stress and depression—as related to lack or loss of wealth—can become debilitating and overwhelming to the body.[44, 49, 50] A person who is able to psychologically adapt to the loss of wealth may have better health outcomes!

Researchers have also sought to understand if absolute wealth and relative wealth have different outcomes on health. Absolute wealth is the minimum amount of income needed to survive; relative wealth is the amount of income a person has compared to others. It could be very discomforting to live with an income that is below the poverty level. However, living at the poverty level would be even more bothersome if someone with similar skills, experience, education, and seniority has a higher salary than you do.

Indeed, several studies have pointed to relative wealth as the main cause of disease or death.[4, 39, 40, 48, 51, 52] An example is in a study of over eight thousand men and women who were followed over time to determine the relationship between wealth and premature death.[34] First, the study confirmed what was already known: that people with low socioeconomic status (SES) had higher death rates than those with high SES. Second, the study included new findings: When people with low SES were grouped by neighborhood (low, medium, and high income), adults who had low SES and lived in high SES neighborhoods had higher mortality rates than the other two groups! A reason for this finding is that the difference between an individual's social position compared to others in his or her community may influence the mortality rate. The fact that relative wealth (rather than absolute wealth) is more troublesome once again highlights the effects of the mind on the body. The lack of material resources was not the cause of distress. Distress was caused by comparing one's material resources to those who have more.

Everything in Moderation

As discussed before, it is important to maintain a balanced state among the four necessities. The paucity or excess of any one necessity may be harmful to a person. Let's explore this in relation to wealth.

It is possible to be a workaholic, overworking yourself to attain a great deal of wealth. However, this excessive work can be harmful. Overworking oneself may come at the expense of your health (a strenuous work schedule can affect physical and emotional health), status (you work so much that it negatively impacts the time spent with your family), and sleep (you don't sleep enough since you are always working).

The accrual of excessive wealth can lead to arrogance or indulgence. For instance, vices and unhealthy pleasures (i.e., illegal drugs, excessive eating, gambling, laziness, and so forth) can result from sudden access to lots of money. At this point, wealth has taken control of your life.

Necessity 4
Basic Drives

Human's basic drives are eating, sleeping, and having sex. These drives are good for well-being when performed moderately and within social norms. Since basic drives are indispensable—we need them to survive and exist on this planet—the affective force's alarm "sounds off" when these drives are threatened. Here's an everyday example of this alarm: Just listen to how much a newborn cries when he or she is hungry, or watch how irritable he or she becomes when sleepy!

In adults, imagine the extreme emotional response of a couple enduring fertility problems or suffering through miscarriages. Procreation (which is essential for human survival) is threatened, and heartbreak occurs. Additionally, it is indisputable that eating, drinking, and sleeping are necessary for our very survival. These are the most instinctual drives too! Adults do not have to think about or remember to eat or sleep. We just satisfy these needs subconsciously when the urge within us demands it. Without food or fluids, individuals perish within days. So it is pretty clear that food and fluids are indispensable to human survival.

As for sleep, rest isn't the only thing that makes a person feel good. A regenerative event that restores and stores away emotional thoughts is required for well-being. This is done through dreaming. Recent advances in electrophysiology and neuroimaging techniques have allowed more in-depth and accurate investigation of sleep. Through these advances, we have learned that brain wave cycles during the day (or while you are awake) are thirty to forty cycles per second. This is very fast! We also know that brain waves are frenetic (or energetic and inconsistent) when you are awake.

Brain waves change when you sleep. During the process of nighttime sleeping, a person normally goes through four sleep stages: three stages of nonrapid eye movements (NREM) and one stage of rapid eye movement (REM).[53] In the first half of the night sleep consists mostly of NREM stages that cycle over ninety-minute periods. During these stages, the brain waves start to slow down to a tempo of two to four cycles per second and become more synchronous.

In the second half of the night, REM sleep prevails. During this stage, the brain waves pick up speed to levels similar to wakefulness (thirty to forty cycles per second) and are frenetic. However, when you are awake your muscles are tense and ready for action. Whereas, in REM sleep your muscles are immobile.

It is during REM that most of a person's dreaming occurs. Think back to a time when perhaps you dreamed of being chased by a threatening animal or person. Despite wanting to escape the threat, you felt like you were moving in slow motion or not moving at all. The reason may be that your body's muscles are paralyzed during REM sleep. (We will discuss the physiology of dreams more in the next chapter.)

It can be said with confidence that the lack of sleep causes premature death. A team of investigators reviewed 101 articles that studied the relationship between sleep and all-cause mortality.[54] (Pooled together, there were 3.5 billion participants and 241,107 cases of all-cause mortality reported.) Compared to the standard of seven hours of sleep per night, a one-hour decrease in sleep was associated with a 6 percent increased risk of mortality due to any cause! Other large studies have found similar findings.[55–57]

As for sex, it is necessary for human existence. Although a person can live very well without sex, humanity itself cannot. Without sex, you and I would not be here! The desire for sex is instinctual and subconscious. However, sexual acts, when done outside the limits of social norms, can lead to serious personal and social consequences. When a person is devoted to one partner and one family, he or she is motivated to protect and build on the family's behalf.

Everything in Moderation

Like the other three necessities, there needs to be a fine balance with the basic drives. Too much or too little is harmful.

Because of the instant pleasures associated with eating, sleeping, and sex, a person may regress to over-indulging when under physical pain or mental stress. When a person feels short-changed in terms of health, status, or wealth, he or she may choose to "make it up" by increasing the fulfillment of the basic drives. Unfortunately, persisting in such practices can lead to unhealthy lifestyles and premature death.

One disease associated with excessive eating—particularly of fats and sugars—is obesity. Obesity is the primary cause of diabetes, hypertension, osteoarthritis, arteriosclerosis, heart disease, strokes, and some cancers.[58] These diseases are the leading cause of death in developed countries.

Excessive sleep is also associated with mortality. Investigators reviewed the literature from around the world to study the relationship between sleep and premature death. This literature review showed that for every hour of sleep above seven hours, the chances of premature death increased by 12 percent.[54] A similar study that reviewed sixty articles from around the world showed that if people slept nine hours, they increased their risk of mortality by 14 percent; if they slept ten hours, they increased their mortality by 30 percent; and if they slept for eleven hours, they increased to 47 percent.[59]

And deviant sex, such as rape and sexual assault, has harmful effects. So too little or too much of the basic drives is not healthy.

We have discussed mostly the psychological and sociological events related to the affective force. Now come the physiological events.

The Buck Stops at the Amygdala

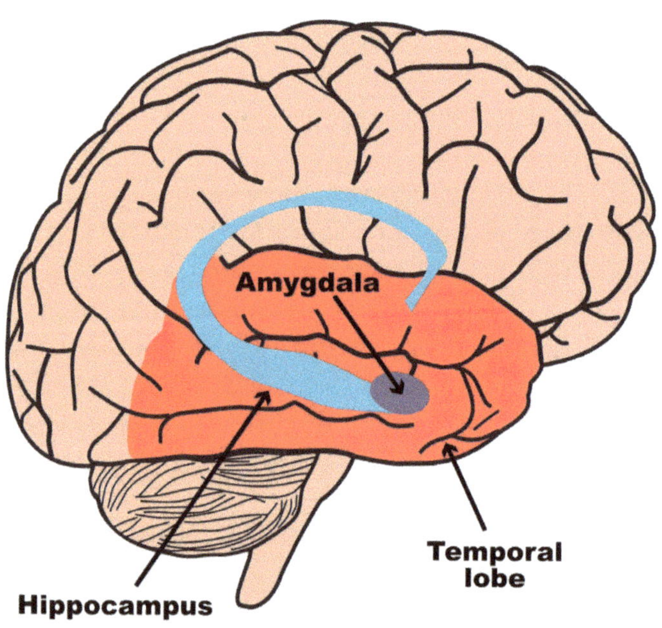

Figure 1. The amygdala

Events that threaten the four necessities will cause activation of the amygdala. The amygdala is the brain processing center of the affective force. We'll talk about why these brain structure is important throughout the rest of this chapter. As you can see in figure 1, the amygdala is a set of almond-shape structures with a cluster of nuclei located in the subcortical region, meaning it is located below the cerebral cortex.

Just how do *unhealthful* events impact the amygdala? French neurosurgeons implanted intracranial electroencephalogram (EEG) electrodes in sixteen brain regions of patients undergoing brain surgery for epilepsy.[60] Intracranial EEG recordings allowed the neurosurgeons to collect the precise activation times of the brain regions with electrodes. Laser stimulations to the brain induced pain in the patients, which the patients postoperatively described as being akin to a "pinprick" or similar feeling. The surgeons recorded the time of the laser stimulation, the time of the brain region activation, and the time of the motor response. The first brain region to trigger an EEG spike was the amygdala! The activation of the amygdala preceded conscious awareness and motor responses by microseconds. The quick response of the amygdala, as caused by unhealthful events, has been reported by other scientists as well.[61–63]

Low *status* triggers amygdala activity[64–66] with several studies indicating childhood neglect leads to exaggerated amygdala reactivity in response to emotional or stressful events.[67, 68] A study conducted by the Max Planck Institute in Germany collected surveys to measure loneliness. They also performed brain MRIs to measure the size of the amygdala in 1,600 participants.[69] This study concluded that higher degrees of loneliness correlated inversely with smaller amygdala volumes. In line with this, a separate study showed that perceived social support was associated with larger amygdala volume.[70] These two studies support the arguments that we will discuss in chapter 4, "Socio-Environmental Force"—that our environmental demands can shape brain structure.

In a study investigating the relationship between *wealth* and the brain, scientists performed brain imaging in response to wealth shocks.[46] Participants had to decide whether or not to accept several gambles presented to them. Based on their decisions, they could win or lose money (a contingent loss). In the same study but another experiment, participants could win or lose money independent of their decision (a random loss). The experiments were performed with the participants lying on their backs while their brains were being scanned using MRI. When participants lost money, irrespective of the experiment, the amygdala was activated on the MRI scans. Other scientists have also shown the amygdala is highly reactive in response to the loss of wealth.[45, 71]

The *basic drives* are under the amygdala's control as well. In animals, when the amygdala is stimulated, it causes increased eating and sexual drives.[65, 72] In humans, when hunger strikes, it is the amygdala that "turns on" the action to satiate the hunger.[65, 72] Sexual cues have also been shown to activate the amygdala in animals and humans.[65, 73, 74]

During sleep, particularly in the REM stage and dreaming, amygdala activation is observed in MRI scans.[75] Dreams are important for two reasons: they encode emotional memories and they tone down emotions. Dreams themselves are emotionally charged and illogical. A person could be dreaming of being chased, ostracized, or ridiculed; losing something of value; or leaving home naked. Yet dreams could also be charged with positive emotions, such as those caused by experiences with sex, friendliness, and wealth attainment.

While one is dreaming, the amygdala, hippocampus, and cerebral cortex have been shown to communicate.[76] If you look at figure 1, you can see that the hippocampus sits right next to the amygdala, and above the amygdala is the cerebral cortex. The hippocampus stores recent memories, typically events that occurred in the last two to three weeks. These memories are stored for a short period of time. When a person is dreaming, the amygdala informs the hippocampus of memories that are important and that need to be transferred to the cerebral cortex. Memories in the cerebral cortex are stored long-term.[75] Thus, dreams perform the function of sorting, filing, and consolidating memories in the synaptic clefts. This process is also called long-term potentiation.

Yet dreams are not exact representations of the actual event. Dreams use symbols to represent real-life experiences. For example, let's say that an employee had a confrontation with his boss. The boss had questioned the employee's productivity. That night the employee dreams of a vicious dog trying to break into his home. In his dream, he is desperately pushing against the door to keep the vicious dog out while the intruder is pushing the door open to see what is inside (the person's home). The dream is symbolic of the boss forcing himself into the employee's workstation to evaluate his productivity. Because the live experience can have an impact on wealth (being fired), the role of the dream is to store this experience in a permanent site. This is done by the amygdala sending a message to the hippocampus to forward the symbolic dream to the cerebral cortex for filing and long-term storage.

Why are dreams so illogical? Why did the employee's dream use the house intrusion as a symbol of a work experience? The reason is that symbols are easier to store and retrieve for future use.

For example, let's say you have your phone carrier return a call to explain an overcharge. The call comes when you are at lunch and are unable to take notes on the conversation. How can you remember the necessary details? Well, here's a trick. Let's say someone named George Jimenez calls first, and George transfers the call to Gwyn Fuller. The date of the call is January 27. During the call, you are told that the overcharge is due to an excess of phone data. It would be easier for you to memorize this event with symbols.[77] Here are some symbols that could represent the actual experience and make it more memorable: George of the Jungle went to the funeral of Janis Joplin who died from an excess of drugs at the age of 27. (George Jimenez is George of the Jungle. Gwyn Fuller went to the funeral. Janis, age 27, is January 27. Excess drugs mean excess data.) It is illogical! But it works, doesn't it?

The second function of sleep, and particularly dreams, is to tone down undesirable emotions.[53] People who lack sleep may never be able to transfer undesirable memories from the hippocampus to the cerebral cortex. If these undesirable emotions stay in the hippocampus, which is close to the amygdala, they will continue irritating the amygdala and cause stress to the individual. Thus, a good night's sleep with REMs is important for distancing distressing memories and keeping them away from the amygdala. Remember, REM sleep ships emotional memories from the hippocampus to the cerebral cortex. These distressing memories may not go away for good, but at least they are not sitting adjacent to the amygdala irritating it. When this function of dreams is met, in effect, people tone down emotionally charged experiences.

The Amygdala in Action

Let's now talk about the amygdala's important tools for defending the four necessities: the hypothalamus and the thalamus.

When the amygdala is activated by threats, it presses the accelerator of the hypothalamus (see figure 2). On command, the hypothalamus turns on the autonomous nervous system and endocrine system, and a fight-or-flight response occurs.[78] Each system is responsible for different things. The sympathetic nervous system regulates temperature, sweat, digestion, body water, breathing, heart rate, blood pressure, cardiac output, and muscle tone. The endocrine system regulates the thyroid, adrenal, growth, reproductive, and pituitary glands. When combined, these brain structures are known as the hypothalamic-pituitary-adrenal axis (HPA axis).

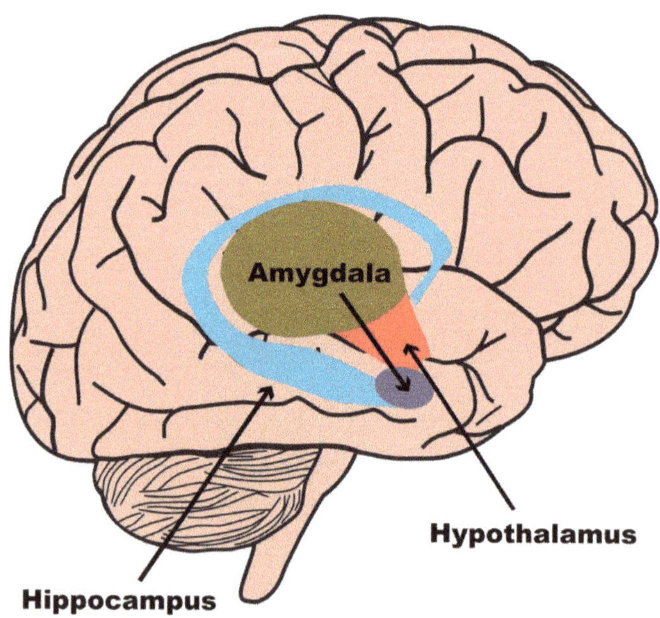

Figure 2. The hypothalamus

Two important hormones controlled by the amygdala via the hypothalamus are adrenaline or epinephrine (nervous system) and cortisol or glucocorticoids (endocrine system). These two hormones are essential in the fight-or-flight defense, but if left uncontrolled through chronic activation, they can affect people adversely and possibly cause early death.

In one study, healthy participants received brain imaging (PET scans) to determine if, over time, amygdala activity was associated with unfavorable health outcomes.[79] After 3.7 years of follow-up on these participants, scientists found that increased amygdala activity was associated with higher inflammation markers and cardiovascular disease. Amygdala activity is also reported to be associated with emotional disorders, such as anxiety and major depression.[61, 80] Like everything else in life, biological organisms must keep themselves in fine balance or homeostasis.

The thalamus and amygdala are the nucleus. They become involved in decision-making when an individual is about to act. The thalamus needs the amygdala to release the fight-or-flight reaction and the amygdala needs the thalamus to project consequences.

The thalamus, along with the cerebral cortex, excels in certain areas. First, they have the capacity to learn from previous experiences. Second, they have the ability to anticipate the consequences of an action.[81, 82] In essence, the amygdala appraises a threat as being either appetitive or aversive while the thalamocortical circuit assesses the threat's magnitude. Third, the thalamocortical circuit can adjust the body's response, so that the amygdala is not reacting on its own. The strategies of appraisal (amygdala) and reappraisal (thalamocortical circuit) allow humans greater use of purposeful reasoning.[83] The thalamus and cerebral cortex, important partners in the amygdala's orbit, will have their own sections in the following chapters.

The Seat for Our Emotions

The seat of emotional processing is the amygdala, which allows a person to feel fear or pleasure. The amygdala-hypothalamus-pituitary circuit produces forty or so brain hormones and neurotransmitters. These hormones and neurotransmitters are responsible for feelings and the body functions that accompany them.

Humans are primarily feeling animals, rather than reasoning animals. Our feelings, which are subconscious, consist of both physical and mental sensations. Feeling hot water is a physical sensation; feeling love is a mental sensation. Emotions are the force that motivates our human behavior. We can be emotional about a number of things, whether we are running to escape a stalker or striving to get into college.

Once the amygdala appraises a stimulus, it works on a strategy for action that travels throughout the entire nervous system. This potential will eventually produce the act itself. This act could vary from a laugh (happy) to a punch (angry).

Be aware that our appraisals can be either automatic or extended.[3] When there is an automatic appraisal, a person will respond subconsciously and in a fraction of a second, to a stimulus. When an extended appraisal occurs, the person will have a conscious response in which the cognitive force (thalamus and cerebral cortex) is brought in for problem-solving. (More on extended appraisals in chapter 2, "Cognitive Force: The Lighthouse.")

What Motivates Us?

Emotions can be motivational. When the environment provokes an emotion there is a motivational force in your body and mind. An emotion occurs when a person perceives something in the environment and then his/her brain makes an emotional judgment about that perception. The judgment will cause the person to act. Notice that reasoning may or may not occur. In fact, it's often skipped.

Let's say that you are walking down the street, and a dog begins to attack you. The emotion you feel starts when you are attacked by the dog. You subconsciously appraise the situation (danger) and quickly climb a tree (the act). As you can see, thinking and reasoning were skipped so that your body could act quickly to keep you safe.

Perception and experience ultimately incite an emotion. In fact, emotions are always intentional because they are caused by something and for something.[3] However, the cause may or may not be real. Emotion could be based on something the person imagines to be true. For example, the stimulus could be "She rolled her eyes at me." And the reality could be she had allergies. Yet while the stimulus (or *presumed* cause) is usually a subjective sensation (she doesn't like me), the object is always objective (that girl).

The cause is also the object when the *presumed* cause is confirmed to be real based on external events and based on observation. To be a *real* cause, it must be observed by others and held up for investigation. Otherwise, the cause will be a fabrication unique to the individual. For example, an employee (the subject) suspects a specific coworker (the object) of stealing (the *presumed* cause) merchandise from the store. The appraisal is negative (anger), the deliberation is reporting to superiors (cognitive), and the behavior is setting up surveillance cameras (act). If the employee is caught with his car's trunk full of stolen merchandise, then the cause also becomes the object.

Emotional circuits, therefore, are built in part around the stimulus and the object and in whole around the individual's perceptions and experiences. What the individual knows and believes ultimately controls what, if any, emotion the individual has.

Correcting Common Misconceptions about Our Emotions

There are some misconceptions about emotions. The common saying "They reacted emotionally" is usually used to indicate that emotions are uncontrollable, negative, and irrational.

Yet emotions may start on a subconscious level, but they end on a conscious level. We recognize and ultimately understand them for what they are. An emotion may start off as a negative response (we are overwhelmed and upset, for example), but we may end up with a positive response (accepting blame and apologizing). Lastly, emotions may start as irrational (wanting to push someone who stepped on your foot) but then become rational ("Don't worry, I'm okay"). Let's explore this in greater detail.

Say that a business owner is busy ordering inventory. Without thinking (subconscious), she bends down to pick up a piece of trash. Farther down the hallway, the business owner encounters a group of employees. She stops to emphasize the importance of customers' first impressions when they walk into the shop (conscious).

Next, let's say that the business owner gets upset because an irate customer is loudly complaining about a valid concern. The business owner gets overwhelmed and upset. But instead of getting angry at the customer, the business owner decides to respond politely and courteously to keep the customer satisfied. Here, the business owner's negative emotion ends up with a positive result.

The third example is how an irrational emotion turns rational. A store manager, without exploring the reasons, gets upset at his employees because sales have decreased for the last three months. The store manager begins researching sales data to compare inventory with items sold. It turns out that the store manager has been ordering items that customers are not buying. An irrational act is rationalized.

The Spectrum of Emotions

We have discussed the energy of emotions. But emotions come in different colors. Emotions consist of a spectrum of attitudes, opinions, passions, moods, and temperaments. Many times, these are used interchangeably and inappropriately.

Attitudes

The short definition of attitude is the disposition a person has toward liking or disliking a stimulus. The long definition of attitude is that it is a mental or neural state of readiness, organized through experience, exerting a directive or dynamic influence upon a person's response to all objects and situations with which the attitude is related.[84] Think about it: An individual is quick to like or dislike a stimulus without giving it all that much thought. When viewed in this way, an attitude is an early segment or only part of an entire emotion.

Here's how attitude and emotion differ:

- An emotion involves stimulus, perception, affection, cognition, and response; an attitude involves stimulus and perception only.
- An emotion is thoughtful; an attitude is reflexive.

- An emotion is in-depth; an attitude is superficial.
- An emotion includes a response; an attitude is only a posture.
- An emotion is a movement; an attitude is a position.

If an attitude's position is neutral, then it does not excite the individual. If the position is one of like or dislike, then the emotion takes it to "the finish line."

Attitudes are important because they provide a narrow window into the affective force. As external manifestations of the affective force, attitudes can be made into psychological concepts that scientists can measure. We measure the position of the affective force through scales that measure attitude (e.g., the Likert scale). For example, a scale may pose the question, "How do you feel about fast-food restaurants? The responses that can then be chosen may be: a) strongly like, b) like, c) neutral, d) dislike, and e) strongly dislike. Although they are indirect and somewhat imprecise, our attitudes are the only tools we have to look into the dark box that is the affective force. The advantage of the Likert scale is that attitudes can be quantified for statistical purposes.

Humans usually have a positive attitude toward the four necessities. However, it is still important to measure people's attitudes toward the necessities since attitudes are built around that person's own unique experiences, culture, and future plans. For example, a plumber and an electrician will have a positive attitude toward wealth but will acquire it through their different personal likes and dislikes. The four necessities are at the heart of the matter, but their learned attitudes are unique dispositions or positions that help them attain the necessities.

The attitudes used to attain the four necessities vary from person to person, and it is this variability that attitudes tend to measure. As you know, attitudes can either be positive or negative. Sometimes even a negative attitude is needed to attain a necessity!

For example, a person with a positive attitude toward exercise and another person with a negative attitude toward processed foods will both likely meet the necessity of health. In a second scenario, one person has a positive attitude toward work. Another person has a negative attitude toward excessive indulgence. Both people will likely attain wealth. In these examples, different people with different attitudes attain the same necessity.

To attain status, a positive attitude toward racial tolerance and/or a negative attitude toward racial discrimination may well allow someone to attain strong relationships. Here we see the phrase "Man you have an attitude" is a misconception. Good attitudes are not only positive. Sometimes negative attitudes are helpful too.

Another common misconception is that attitudes are inborn. Attitudes are learned, so a negative attitude can be changed to a positive attitude by changing our beliefs and knowledge.

Opinions

An opinion is a judgment about an issue or event.[84] An opinion could be considered an attitude because it is a disposition—one that is either positive or negative. An opinion could also fall into the category of beliefs because opinions can be a strong conviction. For example, an opinion is "I think we should limit coal, petrol, and natural gas industries for the sake of controlling climate change." The belief here may be "The emission of large amounts of greenhouse gases is a major cause of climate change."

Other examples of opinions are professional opinions. These come into play, for example, when a patient seeks a second opinion from a medical specialist or a defendant seeks a formal opinion from an attorney.

An opinion is a person's appraisal of the likelihood of an event or object being true, whereas an attitude is a feeling about an event or object. So "The subject of climate change is a hoax" is an opinion. The statement "I like to study climate change" is an attitude.

Public opinion is one example where belief and attitude come together to define opinion. Public opinion surveys and polling are used to measure the shared beliefs and attitudes of a representative sample of a population. (Beliefs, along with knowledge, will be discussed in detail in chapter 2.)

Passions

Passions are the "tail end" of an emotion in the same way that attitudes are the "head end" of an emotion. They are part of a response. Anger, envy, satisfaction, and pride are passions—and responses too.[1] Sometimes there are responses that we desire very much but which we refrain from expressing. For example, we may very much desire to kiss a person whom we find attractive or slap a coworker who has just insulted us, but we do not.

On the other hand, we find it extremely difficult to refrain from expressing our passions in some manner. Fortunately, we only express our passions subtly, even if they are felt intensely. To continue with the same example, although we may not actually try to kiss the attractive person, we may make a facial expression of interest to the other party. And although we may not slap the colleague who has insulted us, we may manifest a facial expression of anger (through a glare or a frown, for example). Our responses here consist of either overt motor responses or subtle passionate expressions.

Passions command specific facial expressions. These expressions are inherited from our primitive ancestors and are transcultural. People from around the world, in all different cultures, manifest embarrassed, ashamed, and ecstatic with similar facial expressions; and it doesn't matter whether they were raised in Europe, Asia, or the United States! And of course, you may not understand the language or behavior of someone from another culture, but if you recognize the person's facial expression, you are then able to read that person's feelings.

Passions may be directed at oneself (inner-directed) or another person (outer-directed). Passions will also vary according to the social norms in which it is expressed. Social morals set the standards of what is "good" behavior. Laws established by society set the rules for what is "good" and "bad" conduct. In turn, a person's passions are defenses that may reflect or show deviations from "the norm."

Generally, there are four types of passions. For instance, deviations from the norm may make a person feel ashamed of himself or herself (*negative inner-directed*). Conversely, if that person exemplifies the norms he or she may feel proud of himself or herself (*posi-*

tive inner-directed). If another person deviates from the norm, then the person observing the act may feel suspicion or hatred toward that other person (*negative outer-directed*). If a person exemplifies the norms, then the person observing the act may feel respect or trust toward that person (*positive outer-directed*). Table 4 offers some examples of common passions, and how they are directed.

Table 4. Popular passions
Positive Inner-Directed
Duty—holding oneself responsible for one's own actions
Ecstatic—a state of overwhelming delight
Happy—demonstrating pleasure
Joy—a feeling of delight
Pride—satisfaction over one's achievements
Positive Outer-Directed
Friendship—favored companionship
Gratitude—thankfulness
Hope—anticipation of a positive fortune
Love—a strong liking or enthusiasm for another person or thing
Satisfied—fulfilled with the outcome
Negative Inner-Directed
Embarrassed—a sense of awkwardness
Guilt—self-reproach for some misdeed
Remorse—accepting responsibility for harm to others
Shame—unfavorable feeling about one's accomplishments or experiences
Shy—feeling timid or bashful
Negative Outer-Directed
Anger—a feeling of extreme hostility
Anguish—an agonizing physical or mental pain
Envy—an ill wanting of something that someone else possesses
Jealous—a feeling of rivalry with another
Sadness—a feeling of loss

Moods

Moods are generalized states of feeling "high" or feeling "low." Being in a good mood produces a "high" feeling and being in a bad mood produces a "low" feeling. Moods are not part of an emotion; they are the aftereffects of the emotion. The emotion ends with a response, and the mood often starts after the response. After an emotion has come and gone, there is usually a mood that lingers for hours (commonly) or days (rarely).

A mood is an unfinished business. A mood may occur if the emotion was incited by a significant stimulus (e.g., a loss, a surprise) or the emotion ended by an inadequate response (e.g., a confrontation occurs, and one is not given time to adequately respond).

Good moods occur when an appetitive or aversive stimulus ends with a positive response; bad moods occur when an appetitive or aversive stimulus ends with a negative response. Here are some examples: A supervisor encounters employees with low morale because of in-fighting (aversive stimulus). The supervisor holds a meeting to handle the situation, and employees end up on good terms by talking with each other (positive response). As a result or aftereffect, the boss finds she is in a good mood for the rest of that day.

Or let's say a salesperson has the opportunity to close a lucrative contract (appetitive stimulus) but errs in the negotiations (negative response). As a result, he remains in a bad mood for several days.

Some people believe that emotions have recognizable antecedents while moods do not, that moods are about "nothing in particular," and that they exist as vague feelings.

Many times, moods are about something or someone. The reality is moods may feel vague because the person doesn't "make the connection" as to why he or she is "feeling this way." This is because the moods are occurring after the emotion has ended and the response has been delivered. There is an appearance of closure. However, if the stimulus was intense (e.g., girlfriend ends a relationship) or the response inadequate (e.g., boyfriend calls but the girlfriend does not pick up), a subconscious feeling of being "high" or "low" lingers. Two weeks later, the boyfriend catches himself in a bad mood but cannot pin down why. If the boyfriend self-reflects enough, he should eventually be able to pin down the cause of the mood. (Most of the time, moods can be discerned through a bit of self-reflection.)

Being "in a mood" also decreases or increases the threshold for future stimuli. For example, if a mother comes home in a bad mood because of a tough day at work, a child crying will easily incite intense emotion. Conversely, if that same person comes home in a good mood because of a fantastic day at work, the child crying may not incite an emotion at all! Because moods set the context for future emotions, moods can subconsciously trigger irrational reactions.

Many times, moods are precipitated by a particular event (as described earlier). But what about when moods have no precipitating event and cannot be explained? Moods, in this case, are caused by neurochemical imbalances. Such imbalances may be short-term or long-term. Short-term neurochemical imbalances are fleeting; they usually last for hours to days and are of no clinical significance. If there is an unexplained mood that lingers for weeks to months, however, then it is an emotional disorder such as major depressive disorder. In this case, medical attention and treatment are needed.

Temperament

Temperament is part of a person's personality. Specifically, temperament deals with emotional dispositions and the intensity and frequency of reactions. For instance, an irritable temperament might make someone more prone to frustration or anger. A calm temperament might mean that a person is slower to react or reacts less intensely. Most behavior scientists agree that temperament is an inherited trait, meaning that it has genetic and biological bases.[85] Scientists believe temperament is inherited because temperamental differences are observed in early development even before environmental factors can have an effect on behavior. More specifically, young humans and animals differ in reactivity (easily irritable) and self-regulation (lack of self-control) to the same stimulus.

The variation in temperament is attributed to the amygdala. Specifically how the amygdala overactivates the hypothalamic-pituitary-adrenocortical axis.[86] Despite most experts agreeing that temperament is an innate trait, a specific gene for temperament has not been found, and the socio-environment can mold and modify how temperament is expressed in children.[87] Furthermore, evidence has shown that a bad temperament in childhood does not necessarily carry over into adulthood.

Summary

The affective force is indispensable for life. It is the defender and first responder of living organisms. The affective force is always on guard appraising incoming stimuli to make sure that the four necessities—health, status, wealth, and basic drives—are not threatened. As important as the affective force is, it can also play tricks in our minds to the point of driving us crazy. On many occasions, events the amygdala considers a threat may be based on fantasy rather than real events. In response to this faulty appraisal, the amygdala will trigger the nervous system to produce stress hormones (corticosteroids and norepinephrine) that elevate blood pressure and blood sugars and cause stomach ulcers and depression.

The control center for the affective force is the amygdala. Events that threaten the four necessities will cause activation in the amygdala as seen in brain imaging studies. Once incited, the amygdala will pull the levers it has at its disposal to increase the heart rate and tighten the muscles to prepare for fight or flight.

The amygdala is the seat of our emotions. An emotion occurs when a person perceives, judges, and acts upon something in the environment. Emotions are motivational. Lastly, attitudes are the "head," passions are the "tail end," and moods are the "aftereffect" of an emotion.

Bibliography

1   Solomon, R. C. *The Passions: Emotions and the Meaning of Life.* 2nd ed. Indianapolis, Indiana: Hackett Publishing Company, 1993.

2   Morrison, S. E., and Salzman, C. D. "Re-valuing the amygdala." *Current Opinion in Neurobiology* 2010; 20 (2): 221–230.

3   Ekman, P., and Davidson, R. J. *The Nature of Emotion: Fundamental Questions.* New York, NY: Oxford University Press, 1994.

4   Kahneman, D. *Thinking Fast and Slow.* 1st ed. New York, NY: Farrar, Strauss, and Giroux, 2011.

5   Ramirez, J. "Suicide: Across the Life Span." *The Nursing Clinics of North America* 2016; 51 (2): 275–286.

6   Bachmann, S. "Epidemiology of Suicide and the Psychiatric Perspective." *International Journal of Environmental Research and Public Health* 2018; 15 (7).

7   Amitai, M., and Apter, A. "Social aspects of suicidal behavior and prevention in early life: a review." *International Journal of Environmental Research and Public Health* 2012; 9 (3): 985–994.

8   Harth, E. *Windows on the Mind: Reflection on the Physical Basis of Consciousness.* New York, NY: William Morrow & Co., 1981.

9   Wasserman, E., Gromisch, D. S., Mixter, R. W., and Lerner, M. *Survey of Clinical Pediatrics.* 7th ed. New York, NY: McGraw-Hill, 1982.

10 Krause, N. M., and Jay, G. M. "What do global self-rated health items measure?" *Med Care* 1994; 32 (9): 930–942.

11 Kaplan, G. A., and Camacho, T. "Perceived health and mortality: a nine-year follow-up of the human population laboratory cohort." *American Journal of Epidemiology* 1983; 117 (3): 292–304.

12 Wannamethee, G., and Shaper, A. G. "Self-assessment of health status and mortality in middle-aged British men." *International Journal of Epidemiology* 1991; 20 (1): 239–245.

13 Lu, Y., Hajifathalian, K., Ezzati, M., Woodward, M., Rimm, E. B., and Danaei, G. "Metabolic mediators of the effects of body-mass index, overweight, and obesity on coronary heart disease and stroke: a pooled analysis of 97 prospective cohorts with 1.8 million participants." *Lancet (London, England)* 2014; 383 (9921): 970–983.

14 Danaei, G., Finucane, M. M., Lu, Y., et al. « National, regional, and global trends in fasting plasma glucose and diabetes prevalence since 1980: systematic analysis of health examination surveys and epidemiological

studies with 370 country-years and 2.7 million participants." *Lancet (London, England)* 2011; 378 (9785): 31–40.

[15] Zong, G., Zhang, Z., Yang, Q., Wu, H., Hu, F. B., and Sun, Q. "Total and regional adiposity measured by dual-energy X-ray absorptiometry and mortality in NHANES 1999–2006." *Obesity (Silver Spring, Md)* 2016; 24 (11): 2414–2421.

[16] Nimptsch, K., and Pischon, T. "Obesity Biomarkers, Metabolism and Risk of Cancer: An Epidemiological Perspective." *Recent Results in Cancer Research Fortschritte der Krebsforschung Progres dans les recherches sur le cancer* 2016; 208: 199–217.

[17] Miell, D., and Dallos, R. *Social Interaction and Personal Relationships.* Thousand Oaks, CA: The Open University, Sage Publication, 1996.

[18] Fuchs, A., Mohler, E., Reck, C., Resch, F., and Kaess, M. "The Early Mother-to-Child Bond and Its Unique Prospective Contribution to Child Behavior Evaluated by Mothers and Teachers." *Psychopathology* 2016; 49 (4): 211–216.

[19] Mogi, K., Nagasawa, M., and Kikusui, T. "Developmental consequences and biological significance of mother-infant bonding." *Progress in Neuro-Psychopharmacology & Biological Psychiatry* 2011; 35 (5): 1232–1241.

[20] Dhand, A., White, C. C., Johnson, C., Xia, Z., and De Jager, P. L. "A scalable online tool for quantitative social network assessment reveals potentially modifiable social environmental risks." *Nature Communications* 2018; 9 (1): 3930.

[21] Cornwell, E. Y., and Waite, L. J. "Measuring social isolation among older adults using multiple indicators from the NSHAP study." *The Journals of Gerontology Series B, Psychological Sciences and Social Sciences* 2009; 64 Suppl. 1: i38–46.

[22] LeRoy, A. S., Murdock, K. W., Jaremka, L. M., Loya, A., and Fagundes, C. P. "Loneliness predicts self-reported cold symptoms after a viral challenge." *Health Psychology: Official Journal of the Division of Health Psychology, American Psychological Association* 2017; 36 (5): 512–520.

[23] Holt-Lunstad, J., Smith, T. B., Baker, M., Harris, T., and Stephenson, D. "Loneliness and social isolation as risk factors for mortality: a meta-analytic review." *Perspectives on Psychological Science: a journal of the Association for Psychological Science* 2015; 10 (2): 227–237.

[24] Steptoe, A., and Kivimaki, M. "Stress and cardiovascular disease: an update on current knowledge." *Annual Review of Public Health* 2013; 34: 337–354.

25 Leigh-Hunt, N., Bagguley, D., Bash, K., et al. "An overview of systematic reviews on the public health consequences of social isolation and loneliness." *Public Health* 2017; 152: 157–171.

26 Adler, N. E., Boyce, W. T., Chesney, M. A., Folkman, S., and Syme, S. L. "Socioeconomic inequalities in health. No easy solution." *JAMA* 1993; 269 (24): 3140–3145.

27 Farah, M. J. "The Neuroscience of Socioeconomic Status: Correlates, Causes, and Consequences." *Neuron* 2017; 96 (1): 56–71.

28 Saydah, S., and Lochner, K. "Socioeconomic status and risk of diabetes-related mortality in the U.S." *Public Health Reports (Washington, DC: 1974)* 2010; 125 (3): 377–388.

29 Mari-Dell'Olmo, M., Gotsens, M., Palencia, L., et al. "Socioeconomic inequalities in cause-specific mortality in 15 European cities." *Journal of Epidemiology and Community Health* 2015; 69 (5): 432–441.

30 Palafox, B., McKee, M., Balabanova, D., et al. "Wealth and cardiovascular health: a cross-sectional study of wealth-related inequalities in the awareness, treatment and control of hypertension in high-, middle- and low-income countries." *International Journal for Equity in Health* 2016; 15 (1): 199.

31 Brinda, E. M., Rajkumar, A. P., Attermann, J., Gerdtham, U. G., Enemark, U., and Jacob, K. S. "Health, Social, and Economic Variables Associated with Depression Among Older People in Low and Middle Income Countries: World Health Organization Study on Global AGEing and Adult Health." *The American Journal of Geriatric Psychiatry: Official Journal of the American Association for Geriatric Psychiatry* 2016; 24 (12): 1196–1208.

32 Boscoe, F. P., Henry, K. A., Sherman, R. L., and Johnson, C. J. "The relationship between cancer incidence, stage and poverty in the United States." *International Journal of Cancer* 2016; 139 (3): 607–612.

33 Andersen, W. S., Blot, W. J., Shu, X. O., et al. "Associations Between Neighborhood Environment, Health Behaviors, and Mortality." *American Journal of Preventive Medicine* 2018; 54 (1): 87–95.

34 Winkleby, M., Cubbin, C., and Ahn, D. "Effect of cross-level interaction between individual and neighborhood socioeconomic status on adult mortality rates." *Am J Public Health* 2006; 96 (12): 2145–2153.

35 Backlund, E., Rowe, G., Lynch, J., Wolfson, M. C., Kaplan, G. A., and Sorlie, P. D. "Income inequality and mortality: a multilevel prospective study of 521 248 individuals in 50 US states." *International Journal of Epidemiology* 2007; 36 (3): 590–596.

36 Crimmins, E. M., Kim, J. K., and Seeman, T. E. "Poverty and biological risk: the earlier 'aging' of the poor." *The Journals of Gerontology Series A, Biological Sciences and Medical Sciences* 2009; 64 (2): 286–292.

37 Mode, N. A., Evans, M. K., and Zonderman, A. B. "Race, Neighborhood Economic Status, Income Inequality and Mortality." *PloS One* 2016; 11 (5): e0154535.

38 Chetty, R., Stepner, M., Abraham, S., et al. "The Association Between Income and Life Expectancy in the United States, 2001–2014." *JAMA* 2016; 315 (16): 1750–1766.

39 Deaton, A. "Policy implications of the gradient of health and wealth." *Health Affairs (Project Hope)* 2002; 21 (2): 13–30.

40 Singh, G. K., and Siahpush, M. "Widening socioeconomic inequalities in US life expectancy, 1980–2000." *International Journal of Epidemiology* 2006; 35 (4): 969–979.

41 Wilkinson, R. G., and Pickett, K. E. "Income inequality and socioeconomic gradients in mortality." *Am J Public Health* 2008; 98 (4): 699–704.

42 Khullar, D. "Health, income, and poverty: where we are and what could help." *Health Affairs Health Policy Brief* (2018). DOI: 10.1377/hpb20180817.901935.

43 Pool, L. R., Burgard, S. A., Needham, B. L., Elliott, M. R., Langa, K. M., and Mendes de Leon, C. F. "Association of a Negative Wealth Shock With All-Cause Mortality in Middle-aged and Older Adults in the United States." *JAMA* 2018; 319 (13): 1341–1350.

44 McInerney, M., Mellor, J. M., and Nicholas, L. H. "Recession depression: mental health effects of the 2008 stock market crash." *Journal of Health Economics* 2013; 32 (6): 1090–1104.

45 Boen, C., Yang, Y. C. "The physiological impacts of wealth shocks in late life: Evidence from the Great Recession." *Social Science & Medicine (1982)* 2016; 150: 221–230.

46 Pammi, V. S. C., Ruiz, S., Lee, S., Noussair, C. N., and Sitaram, R. "The Effect of Wealth Shocks on Loss Aversion: Behavior and Neural Correlates." *Frontiers in Neuroscience* 2017; 11: 237.

47 Marcus, A. F., Echeverria, S. E., Holland, B. K., Abraido-Lanza, A. F., and Passannante, M. R. « The joint contribution of neighborhood poverty and social integration to mortality risk in the United States." *Annals of Epidemiology.* 2016; 26(4): 261–266.

48 Lynch, J. W., Smith, G. D., Kaplan, G. A., and House, J. S. "Income inequality and mortality: importance to health of individual income,

psychosocial environment, or material conditions." *BMJ (Clinical Research Ed)* 2000; 320 (7243): 1200–1204.

[49] Schneiderman, N., Ironson, G., and Siegel, S. D. "Stress and health: psychological, behavioral, and biological determinants." *Annual Review of Clinical Psychology* 2005; 1: 607–628.

[50] Rabkin, J. G., and Struening, E. L. "Life events, stress, and illness." *Science* 1976; 194: 1013–1020.

[51] Fritzell, J., Rehnberg, J., Bacchus Hertzman, J., and Blomgren, J. "Absolute or relative? A comparative analysis of the relationship between poverty and mortality." *International Journal of Public Health* 2015; 60 (1): 101–110.

[52] Wilkinson, R. G. "Socioeconomic determinants of health. Health inequalities: relative or absolute material standards?" *BMJ (Clinical Research Ed)* 1997; 314 (7080): 591–595.

[53] Walker, M. *Why We Sleep: Unlocking the Power of Sleep and Dreams.* New York, NY: Simon & Schuster, 2018.

[54] Yin, J., Jin, X., Shan, Z., et al. "Relationship of Sleep Duration With All-Cause Mortality and Cardiovascular Events: A Systematic Review and Dose-Response Meta-Analysis of Prospective Cohort Studies." *Journal of the American Heart Association* 2017; 6 (9).

[55] Xiao, Q., Keadle, S. K., Hollenbeck, A. R., and Matthews, C. E. "Sleep duration and total and cause-specific mortality in a large US cohort: interrelationships with physical activity, sedentary behavior, and body mass index." *American Journal of Epidemiology* 2014; 180 (10): 997–1006.

[56] Magee, C. A., Holliday, E. G., Attia, J., Kritharides, L., and Banks, E. "Investigation of the relationship between sleep duration, all-cause mortality, and preexisting disease." *Sleep Medicine* 2013; 14 (7): 591–596.

[57] Garde, A. H., Hansen, A. M., Holtermann, A., Gyntelberg, F., and Suadicani, P. "Sleep duration and ischemic heart disease and all-cause mortality: prospective cohort study on effects of tranquilizers/hypnotics and perceived stress." *Scandinavian Journal of Work, Environment & Health* 2013; 39 (6): 550–558.

[58] Trevino, R. P., Pina, C., Fuentes, J. C., and Nunez, M. "Evaluation of Medicare's Intensive Behavioral Therapy for Obesity: the BieneStar Experience." *American Journal of Preventive Medicine* 2018; 54 (4): 497–502.

59 Kwok, C. S., Kontopantelis, E., Kuligowski, G., et al. "Self-Reported Sleep Duration and Quality and Cardiovascular Disease and Mortality: A Dose-Response Meta-Analysis." *Journal of the American Heart Association* 2018; 7 (15): e008552.

60 Bastuji, H., Frot, M., Perchet, C., Magnin, M., and Garcia-Larrea, L. Pain networks from the inside: Spatiotemporal analysis of brain responses leading from nociception to conscious perception. *Human brain mapping.* 2016; 37 (12): 4301–4315.

61 Whalen, P. J., Shin, L. M., Somerville, L. H., McLean, A. A., and Kim, H. "Functional neuroimaging studies of the amygdala in depression." *Seminars in Clinical Neuropsychiatry* 2002; 7 (4): 234–242.

62 Mears, D., and Pollard, H. B. "Network science and the human brain: Using graph theory to understand the brain and one of its hubs, the amygdala, in health and disease." *Journal of Neuroscience Research* 2016; 94 (6): 590–605.

63 Prager, E. M., Bergstrom, H. C., Wynn, G. H., and Braga, M. F. "The basolateral amygdala gamma-aminobutyric acidergic system in health and disease. *Journal of Neuroscience Research* 2016; 94 (6): 548–567.

64 Cacioppo, S., Capitanio, J. P., and Cacioppo, J. T. "Toward a neurology of loneliness." *Psychological Bulletin* 2014; 140 (6): 1464–1504.

65 Berridge, K. C., and Kringelbach, M. L. "Pleasure systems in the brain." *Neuron* 2015; 86 (3): 646–664.

66 Tottenham, N. "Social scaffolding of human amygdala-mPFCcircuit development." *Social Neuroscience* 2015; 10 (5): 489–499.

67 Banihashemi, L., Sheu, L. K., Midei, A. J., and Gianaros, P. J. "Childhood physical abuse predicts stressor-evoked activity within central visceral control regions." *Social Cognitive and Affective Neuroscience* 2015; 10 (4): 474–485.

68 Dannlowski, U., Kugel, H., Huber, F., et al. "Childhood maltreatment is associated with an automatic negative emotion processing bias in the amygdala." *Human Brain Mapping* 2013; 34 (11): 2899–2909.

69 Duzel, S., Drewelies, J., Gerstorf, D., et al. "Structural Brain Correlates of Loneliness among Older Adults." *Scientific Reports* 2019; 9 (1): 13569.

70 Sato, W., Kochiyama, T., Kubota, Y., et al. "The association between perceived social support and amygdala structure." *Neuropsychologia* 2016; 85: 237–244.

71 Aiello, A. E., and Kaplan, G. A. "Socioeconomic position and inflammatory and immune biomarkers of cardiovascular disease:

applications to the Panel Study of Income Dynamics." *Biodemography and Social Biology* 2019; 55 (2): 178–205.

[72] Guyton, A. C., and Hall, J. E. *Textbook of Medical Physiology.* 9th ed. Philadelphia, PA: W. B. Saunders Company, 1996.

[73] Georgiadis, J. R., and Kringelbach, M. L. "The human sexual response cycle: brain imaging evidence linking sex to other pleasures." *Progress in Neurobiology* 2012; 98 (1): 49–81.

[74] Childress, A. R., Ehrman, R. N., Wang, Z., et al. "Prelude to passion: limbic activation by 'unseen' drug and sexual cues." *PloS One* 2008; 3 (1): e1506.

[75] Cipolli, C., Ferrara, M., De Gennaro, L., and Plazzi, G. "Beyond the neuropsychology of dreaming: Insights into the neural basis of dreaming with new techniques of sleep recording and analysis." *Sleep Medicine Reviews* 2017; 35: 8–20.

[76] Bocchio, M., Nabavi, S., and Capogna, M. "Synaptic Plasticity, Engrams, and Network Oscillations in Amygdala Circuits for Storage and Retrieval of Emotional Memories." *Neuron* 2017; 94 (4): 731–743.

[77] Lorayne, H., and Lucas, J. *The Memory Book: The Classic Guide to Improving Your Memory at Work, at School and at Play.* New York, NY: The Random House Publishing Group, 1974.

[78] Kandel, E. R., Schwartz, J. H., and Jessell, T. M. *Essentials of Neural Science and Behavior.* Stamford, CT: Appleton & Lange, 1995.

[79] Tawakol, A., Ishai, A., Takx, R. A., et al. "Relation between resting amygdalar activity and cardiovascular events: a longitudinal and cohort study." *Lancet (London, England)* 2017; 389 (10071): 834–845.

[80] Helm, K., Viol, K., Weiger, T. M., et al. "Neuronal connectivity in major depressive disorder: a systematic review." *Neuropsychiatric Disease and Treatment* 2018; 14: 2715–2737.

[81] Davidson, R. J. "Anxiety and affective style: role of prefrontal cortex and amygdala." *Biological Psychiatry* 2002; 51 (1): 68–80.

[82] Janak, P. H., and Tye, K. M. "From circuits to behaviour in the amygdala." *Nature* 2015; 517 (7534): 284–292.

[83] Feinberg, M., Willer, R., Antonenko, O., and John, O. P. "Liberating reason from the passions: overriding intuitionist moral judgments through emotion reappraisal." *Psychological Science* 2012; 23 (7): 788–795.

[84] Oskamp, S. *Attitudes and Opinions.* 2nd ed. Englewood, NJ: Prentice Hall, 1991.

85 Cassiano, R. G. M., Gaspardo, C. M., and Linhares, M. B. M. "Temperament moderated by neonatal factors predicted behavioral problems in childhood: A prospective longitudinal study." *Early Human Development* 2019; 135: 37–43.

86 Qiu, X., Martin, G. B., and Blache, D. "Gene polymorphisms associated with temperament." *Journal of Neurogenetics* 2017; 31 (1–2): 1–16.

87 Nielsen, J. D., Olino, T. M., Dyson, M. W., and Klein, D. N. "Reactive and Regulatory Temperament: Longitudinal Associations with Internalizing and Externalizing Symptoms through Childhood." *Journal of Abnormal Child Psychology* 2019.

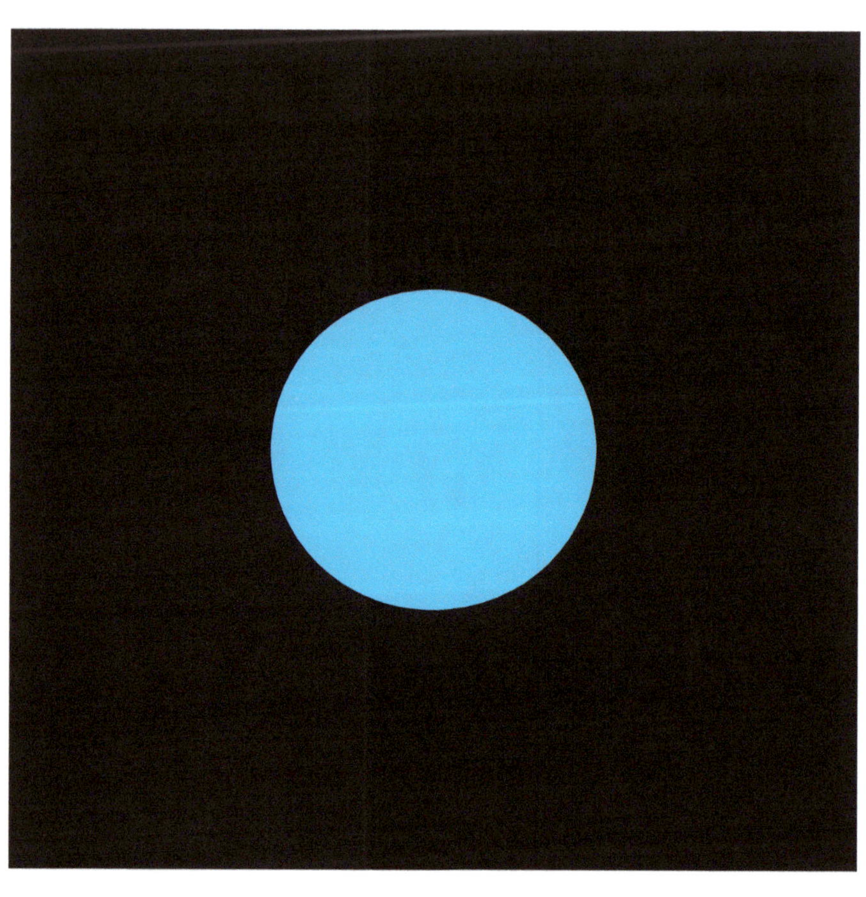

CHAPTER 2

Cognitive Force
The Lighthouse

The purpose of a human's cognitive force is to memorize and reason. Memory is about remembering and recollection of the information that is being stored in the brain. Our reasoning faculty takes that information to comprehend, deliberate, decide upon a specific plan of action, and estimate an outcome. Working memory and reasoning, or intelligence, make up our ability to learn from and grasp our past experiences, to make sense of our present observations and experiences, and to estimate the future consequences of behaviors we undertake. Memory plays its role so we can apprehend and learn while reasoning works to understand and estimate the future impact of actions we choose to take.

The cognitive force is a conglomerate of these information-processing parts and uses both memory and reasoning to guide and support the affective force. On many occasions, though, the cognitive force attempts to control the affective force.

Interestingly, however, and even though it is employing intelligence, the cognitive force generally ends up being a weaker force than the affective force. The affective force driven by feelings is part of the limbic brain while the cognitive force driven by reason/judgment is part of the neocortex. This means that often what the affective force requests or demands will win in a "battle" between the two forces. Many times, this happens because of laziness.[1] It takes effort to apply the cognitive force.

Memory

Memory is information that is either stored for future use or retrieved to create a visual image such as an idea to use for sensory and motor responses. Memories are stored in the synapses, and these are ubiquitous throughout the nervous system. Neurons in the brain and peripheral nervous system are connected by synapses. They all communicate with each other through these structural-electro-chemical bridges called the synaptic cleft. A fourth modality of how neurons communicate has been added to the existing methods. This method is ultraweak photon emissions or UPEs.[2, 3]

Due to its high concentration of synapses, the cerebral cortex has the largest memory storage. The cerebral cortex is the random-access memory (RAM) of the brain where most data is stored and retrieved for quick computing, or in human's case, reasoning.

Memories are not stored randomly in the brain but instead stored by category in direct association with other memories of the same type.[4] Our memories are connected to one another by resemblance, contiguity, and causality.[5] *Resemblance* is storing memories according to similarities such as the subject of gorillas being stored in the great ape section, *contiguity* is storing memories according to when one item is frequently experienced with the other such as a chair and a table being stored together, and *causality* is storing memories according to cause and effect such as diabetes being stored under obesity.

Every neuron has many synaptic connections on its surface. The space between each synaptic connection is called a cleft (see figure 1). Each of our synaptic clefts stores memories; and by storing memories, the synapses undergo structural, electrical, and chemical changes. Synaptic clefts then are bridged together to let electrochemical and light-based information go on to the next set of neurons. Thus, a synaptic cleft is like a capacitor in an electronic circuit.[6] A capacitor is made up of two metallic plates that face each other. And like a synaptic cleft, the capacitor stores energy in an electronic field (See figure 2).

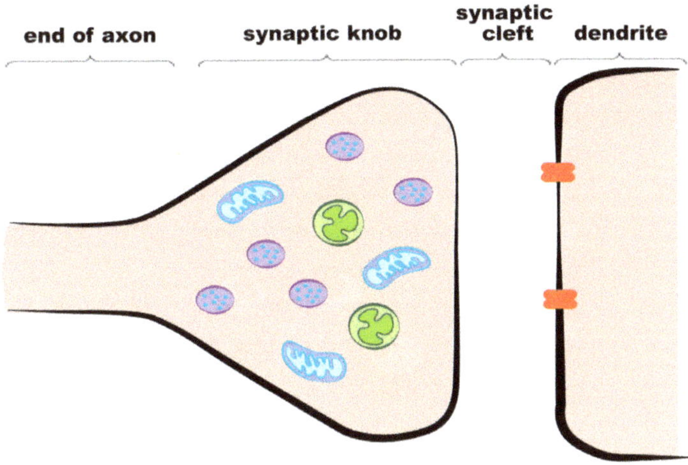

Figure 1. Synaptic cleft

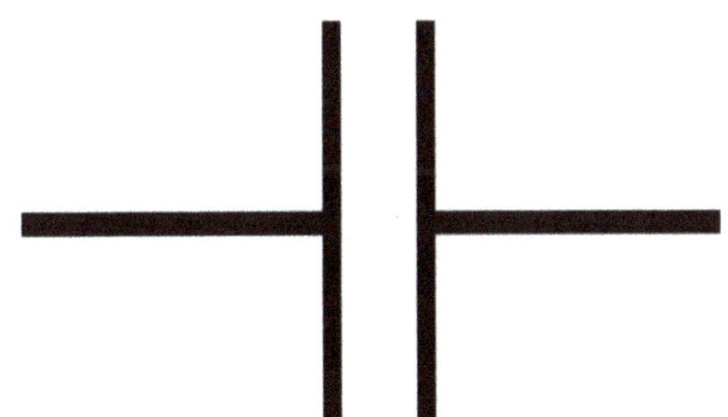

Figure 2. Symbol of a capacitor

Neurons produce streams of UPE and neurotransmitters such as dopamine to communicate.[7–9] The factory within the neuron that produces the UPE is the mitochondria. UPE waves carry energy, but more important, UPE transmits information on how the recipient neurons should respond to the issue in question. It is the importance and frequency of the UPE messages that create structural, chemical, and electrical transformations of the synaptic clefts. Furthermore, UPE activity has been associated with cerebral metabolism, electroencephalogram (EEG), cerebral blood flow, meditation, consciousness, and cognitive processes.

Because of the importance and frequency of UPE messages, synapses are fortified by leaving memory traces or engrams that play a major role in memory. A memory engram is an ensemble of neurons where specific learning experiences are stored in the neuron's synapses.[10] An individual's attitudes, beliefs, knowledge, and behaviors are stored and released by networks of memory engrams. Memory engrams connect and communicate with engrams in other sections of the brain. They determine who we are.

Whether a memory engram remains a short-term one or becomes a long-term one depends on a few things:

- how the information is entered
- how important is the information that is entered
- how aversive is the information
- how often the particular information is used (as those memories not used for a period of time will eventually decay, meaning be forgotten)[11]

Let's explore these points in more detail. In terms of how the information is entered into our brain, those memories created by *extrospection* (an occurring event, such as being attacked by a dog) will enter the clefts with more force and vigor than memories created by *introspection* (just thinking about being attacked by a dog). The importance of entering information affects the length of its storage. Any information that gets, keeps, and increases the four necessities is stored longer than information irrelevant to the individual's four necessities. An electrician, but not the plumber, will remember long-term the new dawn-to-dusk light bulbs that just came out on the market. Aversive information is stored for longer periods of time than appetitive information.[1] For example, pleasant experiences usually leave short-lasting impressions on a person, whereas painful experiences leave long-lasting impressions.

The frequency of information usage impacts memory storage: Habits facilitate synaptic transmissions, whereas inactivity inhibits synaptic transmissions. So each time a particular activity is performed, a signal representing that activity passes across the synaptic cleft. The frequent use of this pathway makes those synapses more capable of transmitting that same signal again and again. This phenomenon is called long-term potentiation, which is the synapses' ability to strengthen in response to increases in their activity, hence solidifying memory. Nonuse of a given synapse or decreases in their use results in long-term depression and loss of that nugget of memory. The innate ability to wire new circuits and rewire lost connections is called *neuroplasticity*, which is defined as the synaptic ability to build new connections. Synapses, therefore, perform a selective action by inhibiting or facilitating the transmission of electrical information through its clefts.

Interestingly, however, whether a person is raised in an enriched or impoverished socio-environment eventually determines whether his or her synaptic structural, electrical, and chemical changes will be overdeveloped or underdeveloped (respectively). Specifically, studies have shown that animals raised in larger cages with more physical activity devices have stronger synaptic clefts than animals raised in smaller cages with no physical devices.[12, 13] So being raised in an impoverished socio-environment may be a more important factor than innate abilities in explaining why some people under develop neuroplasticity.[14] Neuroplasticity strengthens synapses.

Memorable Categorization and Filling

In the "grand scheme" of memory, memory is divided into two large categories: *declarative* (knowing *what* something is) and *nondeclarative* (knowing *how* to do something).[15] Declarative memory is the recollection of events, facts, and concepts. Nondeclarative memory is the performance of skills, tasks, and habits, as well as the ability to remember the location or position of places and objects.

The recollection of events is further known as *episodic memory* and the recollection of facts and concepts as *semantic memory*. The performance of skills, tasks, and habits is further known as *procedural memory* and the ability to locate sites and objects as *spatial memory*.

The process of filing declarative memories occurs in two phases. To fully grasp this method, let's use the following case scenario as an example. Imagine an architect designing a high-rise building. The architect researches and collects the literature she needs to design and construct the building. She then spreads the reviewed literature, consisting of sixty to seventy articles, over a table. Once the architect categorizes these articles by "design" and "construction" subjects, she stores them in the corresponding sections in a filing cabinet. When she needs them again, she will know where to quickly find them.

If we apply this example to the filing of our memories, the hippocampus is like a table on which lies a host of unorganized articles, and the cerebral cortex is the filing cabinet in which the articles are sorted by subject matter before they are actually stored.[16] Now if we simply "dumped" all our memories into the cerebral cortex without imposing any organization on them, the thalamus (see below) will lose valuable time looking for a particular memory each time it is needed. Life would then become chaotic and disorganized indeed if we couldn't easily "find" what we already had known!

Making Memories More Permanent

In chapter 1, I discussed how sleep, particularly REM sleep, was important to transferring emotional memories from a temporary site (the hippocampus) to a more permanent site (the cerebral cortex). However, while emotional memories (nondeclarative) are stored during REM, factual and conceptual (declarative) memories are stored during non-REM sleep.[17, 18] But like everything in science, nothing is written in stone. While you may find seven studies supporting the association of non-REM sleep with declarative memories, there are another three that do not.[19]

As mentioned in chapter 1, REM sleep is characterized by fast and frenetic brain waves, and non-REM sleep or delta wave sleep by slow brain waves. The burst of activity between the thalamocortical tract during slow-wave sleep has been shown to consolidate memories from temporary to permanent sites in the cerebral cortex.[20] This shows the beneficial role of a good night's sleep in preventing memory loss, although even memory stored in the permanent site will ultimately be lost if left unused.

Reasoning

The purpose of reasoning is to take a person's thoughts and create ideas from them. To make a computer analogy, memories are information bits (basic computing units), and thoughts are information bytes (8 bits in a byte). Several memories make up a thought. The role of reason is to deliberate among the many thoughts that flash through our mind so we may formulate an idea. Our thoughts are our mental processes, and our ideas are our plans or strategies that can come from these thoughts. In essence, thinking is a long-acting thought. It can keep going on and on in the mind unabated!

How we decide whether to switch or stay in the same lane on the road is a simple example of the ability to reason. For example, a man driving on the highway is stuck behind a lot of traffic in the right lane. He reasons that the entrance ramp ahead will further slow down traffic in the right lane, so he formulates a strategy to avoid being stuck in traffic. He will move into the left lane. But then he observes that the 18-wheeler up ahead in the left lane is slowing down the cars behind it. So he formulates a second strategy—stay in the right lane. In this case, he is using his reasoning to estimate the best response based on past memories, present observations, and future consequences. Reasoning may not always reach or come to the absolute truth, but it will reach a probability (*verisimilitude*).

Reasoning consists of neurons interacting from one memory to another until the person makes a decision (*syllogistic reasoning*).[21] Reasoning happens by the neurons networking with one another via synapses, and one single neuron on its own is never enough to incite a response. Instead, reason must round up an ensemble of neurons to form a pathway of synaptic bridges toward a decision. A term used for this roundup is *coherence*. Coherence means that the UPE waves released by neurons organized themselves into an interconnected system working as a synchronic electromagnetic field.[7]

When deciding on a plan or an action/behavior, neuronal "pools" come to a consensus by summing up the votes (signals) from each single neuron. This process, called *summation*, decides the direction a person's action takes. Neurons also question and oppose one another, and those equipped with the most knowledge usually rule (*scientific reasoning*).

An Individual Act

To act is to perform a behavior. An act is the choice of an individual. All acts are a matter of choice, and only the individual—not the socio-environment—decides which acts he or she is going to choose.

Even if a person has been raised, or is presently living, in a difficult and traumatic socio-environment, his or her response to adversity remains a matter of personal choice. A person cannot and should not blame anyone else but him or herself for the actions he or she takes; it all comes down to personal choices. In making his or her own choices, a person can control his or her own destiny.

Of the Two, Which Force Has the Greater Power?

In the process of reasoning and deciding on a modus operandi, it is not unusual for the affective and cognitive forces to disagree. For example, a boss may take disciplinary actions against an employee, and the employee's initial reaction may be to get angry and yell back at the boss (affective force). At the same time, the employee reasons that exhibiting an angry reaction may get him fired, so he weighs the future consequence of being unable to pay his bills if he loses his job (cognitive force). In line with this, while the affective force is quite quick to attack and defend, the cognitive force will attempt to restrain the affective force from attacking or undertaking an action if, chances are, the action taken is going to be followed by an unfavorable outcome (in this example, losing his job).

But there are other instances where the cognitive force may not be successful at restraining the affective force. If, for example, a fire breaks out at a workplace and all the exits are blocked, the affective force may urge the person to jump out a second-floor window to escape while the cognitive force may reason that the outcome will be negative—a broken ankle, perhaps. In this case, though, the affective force will overrule the cognitive force because it is a choice between either staying alive with a broken ankle or dying with intact bones.

Fortunately, the two forces are in sync most of the time, which gives way to volition. *Volition* is the power of choice where a person uses his or her will. Volition is an "executive order" to commit to a particular course of action. The cognitive and affective forces evoke volition by presenting their objective to it. Volition allows a person to determine their own inclination toward a particular end once he or she knows the means to reach it. Thus, deliberation (or *readiness potential*) must precede volition.

Thalamus

Just as the amygdala is the brain's processing center of the affective force, the thalamus is the brain's relay station and processing center of the cognitive force. The thalamus sits right above the amygdala and looks like a set of binoculars with its two lobes (see figure 3).

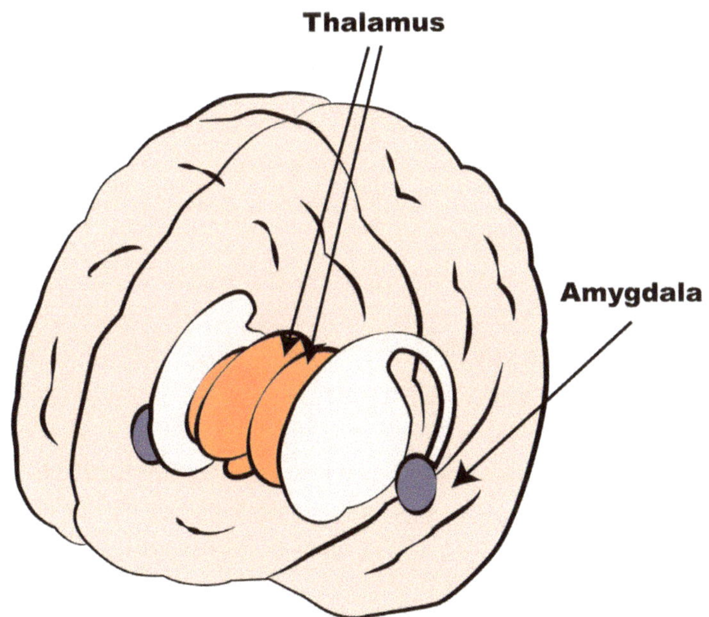

Figure 3. Thalamus

Once it was thought that it was the cerebral cortex that made archaic humans *Homo sapiens*. However, new science shows that it is actually the thalamus that rules.[22] Indeed, the thalamus operates as the "master regulator" of the cerebral cortex. And it might have been the constant demand from the thalamus that made the cerebral cortex—particularly the front part of it—"shape up."

The thalamus is where the external and internal worlds meet to "learn their fate," in the sense of ignoring or giving significance to events. External sensory stimuli—those which are visual, audio, tactile, and taste (all except for smell)—come to the thalamus for a "checkup" or evaluation before being sent up to the cerebral cortex for understanding and reasoning. Similarly, internal stimuli such as ideas coming down from the cerebral cortex go to the thalamus for a checkup as well before they are sent up (again) to the cerebral cortex for further computation. Thus, the thalamus, and not the cerebral cortex, is in the "driver's seat" when it comes to cognitive matters.

Traffic Control

External sensory stimuli that come in from the socio-environment and up to the thalamus are called *first order relays*.[23] Internal stimuli that come down from the cerebral cortex to the thalamus are called *higher order relays*. No matter where the stimuli originate, they come to the thalamus first and then are sent to the cerebral cortex for computation and action.

The connections going through the thalamus, however, are not just relays, or mere "passing-on" of the batons; they have a tremendous influence on *what* and *how much* (if any) goes on up to the cerebral cortex for computation and action. There are some messages that the thalamus does not consider important, so it just lets them "fizzle out."

The thalamus is a complex central station with multiple functions:

- *Pathways*—route information across cortical and subcortical structures
- *Gatekeepers*—function as thresholds to decide which signals should or should not be sent to the cortex

- *Mediators*—gets information from one cortical site and send it on to another cortical site
- *Regulators*—activate some cortical areas, while deactivating others.[24]

Which action to take is based on how the thalamus perceives the stimulus coming from the socio-environment (extrospection) or the thought coming from inside the mind (introspection).

Critical Inputs into the Hard Drive

The cerebral cortex operates in such close association with the thalamus, it can almost be considered a unit of the thalamus,[25] as the thalamus connects to every region of the cerebral cortex (see Figure 4). The thalamus has two types of inputs that it sends up to the cerebral cortex and down to subcortical areas once processing has occurred: drivers and modulators.[26]

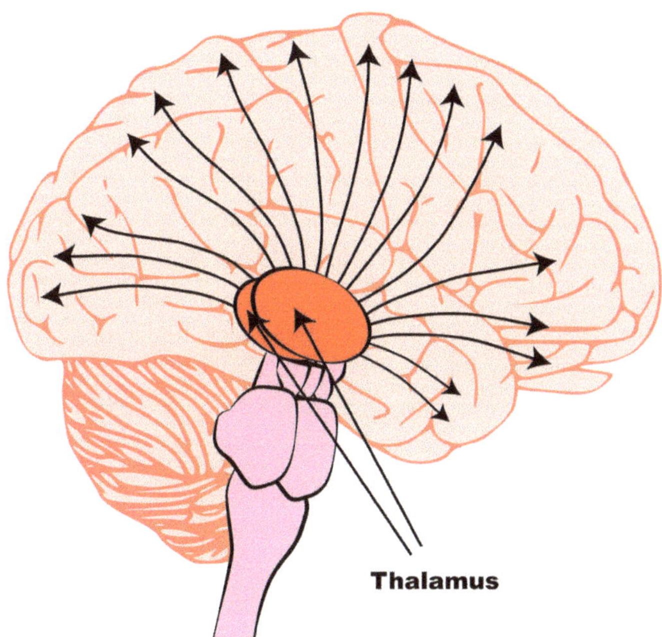

Figure 4. Thalamus connectivity to the cerebral cortex

Drivers comprise the minority (~10%) of the inputs and transmit unaltered signals to the cerebral cortex. Drivers determine the *where*. Driver inputs determine to which ensemble of sensory neurons (the receptive field) a stimulus should be sent for processing. The *receptive field* of a central neuron is defined as the region of the brain's sensory surface which when stimulated by an adequate stimulus, produces an excitatory response. The drivers relay this information "as is" or without modification to the cerebral cortex and supply information about instructions, such as the type of action to take, also to subcortical centers. The instructions are products of the processing (or deliberation) that occurred among a set of neurons.

Modulators form the majority (~90%) of the inputs and transmit altered signals to the cerebral cortex. Modulators determine the *what*. Without ever changing the properties of the receptive field, modulator inputs alter the transmission of sensory-driven activity by influencing how and what driver signals get relayed to the cortex. Modulators influence the transmission by enhancing or attenuating the signal, and modulator inputs also modify how driver inputs are processed in the cerebral cortex.

Thus, we can view the cerebral cortex as playing "second fiddle" to the thalamus. Without thalamic excitation of the cerebral cortex, there is no cortical activity.[25] Nonetheless, the cerebral cortex is still an important instrument for storing memory, as well as for computing, and also for generating movements or actions of the body. (The cerebral cortex's role in language will be discussed in the next chapter.)

The primary function of the cerebral cortex is storage. Envision the cortex's memory function in this way: What hard-drive memory storage is to a computer, the cerebral cortex is to a person's brain. The cerebral cortex has different file cabinets where visual (occipital cortex), auditory (temporal cortex), tactile (parietal cortex), smell (temporal cortex), taste (insular cortex), and motor function (frontal cortex) data are stored. And as mentioned earlier, memories are stored in the synapses. Reports indicate that one synapse corresponds to approximately 4.7 bits of computer memory storage.[27] If the cerebral cortex has an estimated 125 trillion synapses, then the brain storage capacity amounts to 73.44 terabytes—an amazing amount of storage! To provide you with a reference point (or two) for this information: The brain has 1,500 times more synapses than the Milky Way has stars, and one person's brain's memory storage capacity is equivalent to that of 118 desktop hard drives!

The second function of the cerebral cortex is computation. This computational ability can range from processing sensory data to abstract reasoning. For computing to occur, not one but an ensemble of neurons needs to be activated and engaged.[28]

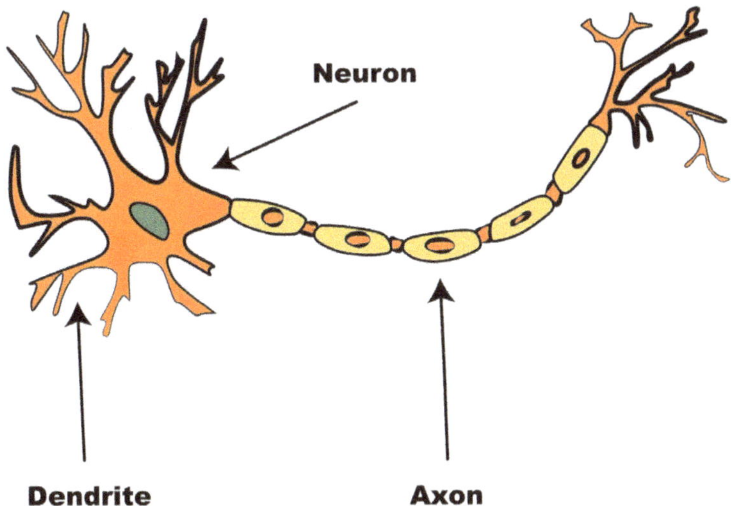

Figure 5. Axons and Dendrites

The cortical regions form different functional neural networks. These neural networks receive and send out patterns of activity through tracts of axons to other cortical areas and the thalamus. (Note figure 5. Axons and dendrites are "arms" that stick out of a neuron. Axons send out and dendrites receive messages among neurons.)

In fact, there is generally frenetic back-and-forth communication between the cerebral cortex regions (the cortico-cortical tracts), as well as among cerebral cortex regions and the thalamus (cortico-thalamic-cortical tracts). With the thalamus as the "transfer node" between the cerebral cortices, it can influence how and what driver messages get related to the cortex, and it can modulate these messages to correspond to the contextual setting that triggered the process of computation.[24] Through this method, the cerebral cortex processes stored letters, words, numbers, and images to recreate meaningful ideas and behaviors. This is *reasoning*.

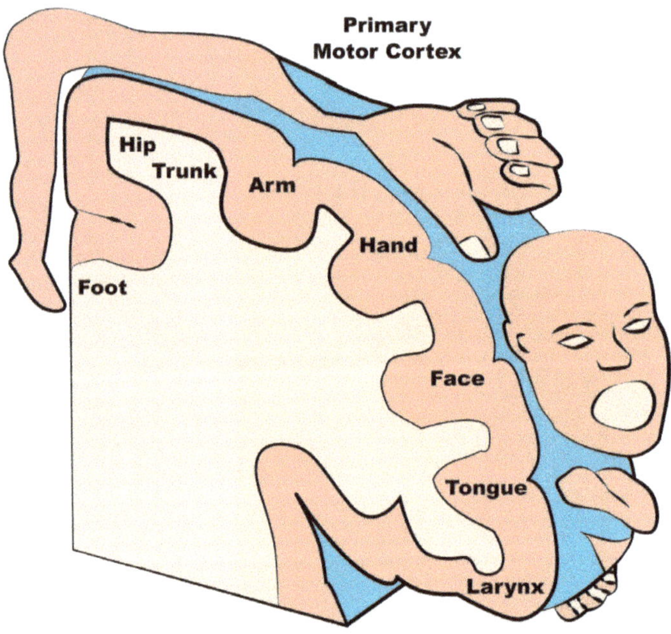

Figure 6. Motor cortex topographical representation

The cerebral cortex's third function is to transform the computations into motor activities. The behaviors that ensue are motor activities or actions that can be observed, such as talking, eating, swallowing, running, crying, and so on. Thus, it makes sense that muscles from every single part of the body have their specific site in the motor cortex.[25]

Figure 6 shows a topographical representation of the different muscles in the cortex. These sites were discovered during neurosurgery when surgeons electrically stimulated different areas of the brain's motor cortex and recorded the muscles that were activated.

It turned out that the body parts that take the most space in the motor cortex are hand and speech muscles, which is not all that surprising given that it was bipedalism and language that made hominids human. The leading theory of how bipedalism evolved suggests that females favored mating with males who could provide for them and their progenitors. To be successful providers, the males required their arms and hands to be free to carry provisions to their female partners.[29] As for language, it speaks for itself. Language enabled social communication, networking, and shared meanings. I will explore the cortex's fourth function—the role of the cerebral cortex in language—in the next chapter.

As for the prefrontal cortex, it is special in many ways. First, it functions in close association with the motor cortex to plan out fine and detailed sequences of motor activities. Many of the resulting outputs from the prefrontal cortex to the motor cortex pass through the thalamus for executive approval.

Second, the prefrontal cortex is also capable of more elaborate computing than the rest of the cerebral cortex[25] and thus is known to be the neurobiological basis of "working memory." What this means is that the prefrontal cortex can track many more bytes of information and recall them, something that is needed for more elaborate thoughts. By combining bytes of information, the prefrontal cortex can weigh options, consider consequences, solve problems, and keep humans grounded in societal norms, laws, and moral standards. The products of these bytes of information are beliefs and knowledge (to be discussed in the next section).

Tied to the Amygdala

Earlier I mentioned that the actual execution of any potential motor activity needs to pass by the thalamus for "appraisal and approval." But to enact a behavior, "the buck does not stop" with the thalamus. The thalamus and amygdala work in conjunction within the brain and the neural pathways connecting both are strong (See Figure 7).

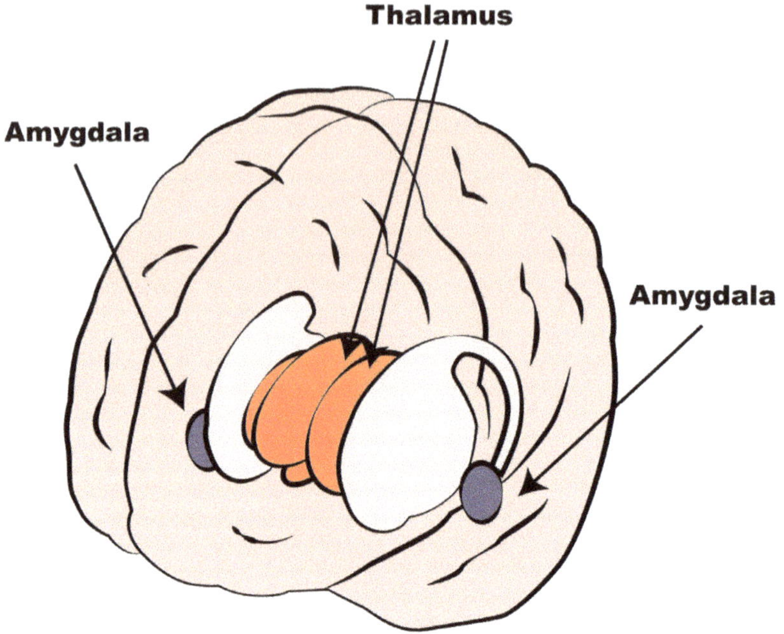

Figure 7. Thalamus-amygdala nucleus

By this I mean the decision of what, when, and how to execute a motor activity becomes a matter of discussion between the thalamus and amygdala; and many times they do not agree! As stated earlier, the affective force is a stronger force than the cognitive force because it is the first responder and it deals with a person's immediate survival; the cognitive force can be quite a persuasive force via computation and estimation. Another contribution of the thalamus is its role as a lighthouse in terms of focusing awareness on someone or something. As mentioned on several occasions, many of the amygdala's actions are subconscious. This is not the case with the thalamus. This is explained in the following paragraph.

What and Where Is Consciousness in the Brain?

Consciousness is the state of being awake, and of being aware of the socio-environment and self. Being aware of oneself means that a person can think of what he or she is thinking and reflect on his or her own appearance and behaviors. Nothing else but consciousness can unite remote existences (items and events that really exist) into the same person. The physical body can't do so because a person's organs and tissues degenerate and regenerate daily, making what a person looked as a child markedly different from how he or she looks once an adult. Thus, personal identity is determined by our consciousness of self and others.

While damage to the cerebral cortex has a none-to-little effect on consciousness,[30] damage to the thalamus leads to a loss of consciousness. The anatomy and physiology of the relationship between the thalamus and cerebral cortex imply that the thalamic-cortical tracts play the main role in consciousness.[31, 32] Evidence for this comes to us through the use of anesthesia. Anesthesia causes a loss of consciousness by sundering the connection between the thalamus and the cerebral cortex.[33] The connection between the thalamus and cerebral cortex thus is like a plug connecting to a socket to turn on the light. Humans need both (thalamus and cerebral cortex) to "light up" their consciousness.[34]

Beliefs and Knowledge

What specifically is the information being stored in our memory bank? That information is beliefs and knowledge. *Beliefs* are energetic ideas, and *knowledge* is the evidence that arises from the comparison of ideas. These two kinds of information originate in the socio-environment. The difference between belief and knowledge is a matter of degree, as they are two variants of the same spectrum. Belief is an individual conviction that something is true, whereas knowledge is a universal conviction that something is true. Both are important with only a "gray line" separating the two.

We learn our beliefs and attain knowledge through sensory experiences. (Learning refers to the abstraction of beliefs and knowledge from the socio-environment.) Beliefs and knowledge enter people through their sensory receptors—mostly, the visual and auditory receptors. Thus, beliefs and knowledge leave impressions in the synaptic clefts.

Which is Which?

Beliefs and knowledge arise from cultural practices transmitted from person to person and from generation to generation. To comprehend the difference more clearly between beliefs and knowledge, there is a simple rule some people offer up or follow: If a statement involves more letters than numbers, then the message is a belief, whereas if a statement involves more numbers than letters, then the message is knowledge. In general, literature, philosophy, and fine arts are beliefs; science and math, are knowledge.

To further understand this difference using some everyday examples, if there are two routes to reach a location, a person may *believe* one route is shorter than the other. If a person measures the distance between both routes, then this person *knows* one route is shorter than the other.

Or an employee *believes* that an employer laid him off for personal reasons. If the employer documents the times the employee came in late and the times he handed in projects past due, then the employer *knows* the employee is inefficient. The following are more characteristics that distinguish beliefs from knowledge.

Complementary Dual

Beliefs are hypotheses that stretch the mind;
Knowledge is method that narrows the imagination.
Beliefs transcend life;
Knowledge categorizes it.
Beliefs are mostly taught at home;
Knowledge is mostly taught at schools.
Beliefs are faith;
Knowledge is science.
Beliefs are blue sky;
Knowledge is solid ground.
Beliefs are relative;
Knowledge is absolute.
Beliefs are forethought;

Knowledge is aftermath.
Beliefs are expanding waves;
Knowledge is collapsing particles.
Beliefs are momentum;
Knowledge is position.
Beliefs without knowledge are stagnant;
Knowledge without beliefs has no meaning.
Beliefs and knowledge are energy.
Beliefs and knowledge are spirits.

It's a Matter of Energy

Beliefs and knowledge are energy in the form of UPE that emanates out of an individual to influence not only himself or herself but the socio-environment too. The energy that comes from beliefs and knowledge can change that person as well as his or her socio-environment. Happily, both beliefs and knowledge provide the mechanism for transmitting the energy that they constitute. What the individual believes and knows is what the individual will do!

You may be wondering, "How it is that beliefs and knowledge represent energy, and how and where is this energy stored?" To understand the answer to these questions, it is important to understand the function of capacitors in an electronic circuit. Capacitors store electrical energy (see figure 2 above). Notice how the diagram representing the electronic capacitor looks like the illustration of the synapses, for both have two parallel conductors with a space between them.

Now one capacitor plate has a negative charge and the other a positive charge, and as you might know by now, opposites attract. By attracting each other, the opposing plates with opposite charges produce an electrical field. This electrical field, located between the capacitor plates, represents stored energy.

Similarly, in the synaptic clefts, there are positively charged cations on one side (sodium, potassium, and calcium) and negatively charged anions (chloride) on the other side.[25] Because chloride is the smaller of the ions, it passes through the membrane pore to the other side, whereas the larger ions of sodium, potassium, and calcium stay on the same side. The opposing electrical charge produces an attraction. This space of attraction, or the electrical field, creates a *capacitance* or the ability to store energy.

Now that we understand where beliefs and knowledge are stored in the body, let's explore the energy they have to influence not only us but our social environment. Aspiration, faith, and wisdom are carriers of this energy. Used correctly, humans can cure disease; if used incorrectly, they can lead to the path of destruction. This is explained in the following lines.

How Our Beliefs and Knowledge Influence Us

Aspire

Aspiration is the belief that a person has that he or she can accomplish his or her goals. To aspire is to develop a drive for high achievements (of any kind, really) and to strive toward an end. When a person uses his or her ability to visualize the future, plan ahead, analyze, and calculate various pathways of how to reach a particular goal, he or she is using aspiration.

The ability of aspiration is unique to humans: Animals cannot influence their efforts by self-reflecting on what they can or cannot do. Humans, on the other hand, can generate alternate solutions and evaluate potential outcomes. They are not content with simply satisfying the basics of the four necessities; they tend to increase them.

Since we are capable of aspiring and striving for something beyond immediacy, we are capable of wishing for higher goals and purposes. That sets us apart from the rest of the animal kingdom.

Aspiration and planning are functions of the prefrontal cortex, that part of the brain that differentiates humans from apes. The prefrontal cortex, in conjunction with the thalamus, has the ability to prognosticate and plan for the future. The prefrontal cortex can consider the consequences of motor actions before they are performed and delay the actions until all sensory information is analyzed and outcomes weighed.

Aspiration stands out among the various types of beliefs because it is a strong motivator of behavior. By foreseeing the consequences of their actions, individuals convert perceived future outcomes into present-day motivators of their behaviors.

In fact, aspiration is so strong a motivator that behavior modification theories are using it to design programs to improve health behaviors (see table 1).

Table 1. Terms used instead of aspiration in behavior modification theories[35]		
Term	Definition	Theory
Behavioral beliefs	Beliefs about personal attributes of performing the behavior weighted by evaluations of those outcomes	Theory of reasoned behavior
Expectancy outcomes	Beliefs that a certain course of action will change a targeted outcome	Health belief model
Self-efficacy	Beliefs in one's ability to take action based on anticipated consequences	Social cognitive theory

Faith

Faith is belief and trust in God and/or in the doctrines of a religion. Prayer and meditation belong to the realm of faith. Both are usually forethoughts in the sense that through prayer and meditation, humans usually are projecting their imagination into the future. In both prayer and meditation, people wish for positive events to happen to them and/or to others, seeing that kindness and goodness are the intentions of faith.

Sometimes when we use the word *faith* in daily or conversational usage, we use it to offer hope to someone who is in some sort of distress. For example, when things go wrong, we may console one another by telling the other person to "Have faith!" By telling another "You must have faith," we are attempting to throw them a rope so they can climb out of the "hole" in which they currently are finding themselves. Faith offers them hope, and that hope is directing them toward happiness and a better life.

Faith or Reason

Faith and reason might compete for human attention. But because they are separate and distinct, instead of competing, they have additive effects. The interaction of, and the difference between, faith and reason cannot be better explained than through the words of St. Thomas Aquinas:[36]

> Faith dominates reason, not so much as a mode of knowledge, for it is, on the contrary, an inferior type of knowledge on account of its obscurity, but insofar as it places human thought in possession of an object which reason would be incapable of grasping naturally.
>
> Hence, faith gives rise to a whole series of influences and actions, the consequences of which are of the utmost importance within reason itself, which yet does not cease to be pure reason. Faith in revelation does not result in destroying the rationality of our knowledge, but, on the contrary, in allowing it to develop more completely; just as grace does not destroy our nature, but fertilizes, exalts, and perfects it, so faith, by its influence upon reason as such, promotes the development of a rational activity of a more fruitful kind.

Faith and reason can neither contradict each other, nor ignore each other, nor be confused. Reason may well try to justify faith: it will never transform faith into reason, for as soon as faith were to abandon authority for proof, it would cease to believe; it would know. And faith may well move reason externally or guide it internally; reason will never cease to be itself, for once it renounced the proof of its assertion, it would deny itself and would vanish to make room for faith. It is, therefore, the inalienability of their proper essences which permits them to act upon each other without contaminating each other.

Wisdom

Wisdom is the ability to use one's knowledge and faith to improve oneself and the socio-environment. Thus, wisdom is altruistic in that it benefits others more as well as ourselves. It is the ability to make prudent decisions based on facts and a belief that a certain action will produce a specific outcome.

When we are being wise, we are using our knowledge to improve ourselves, and we also can use that knowledge to improve the life of others and the natural environment

There are two sources of our knowledge: sensible (meaning practical and functional) and understanding (having insight or good judgment).[37] *Sensible knowledge* either is given to a person by the socio-environment or the individual extracts it from the socio-environment. Sensible knowledge enters an individual through his or her sensory receptors (visual, auditory, touch). For example, a person approaches a home, smells a delicious aroma in the area, and sees a pie cooling on the windows, so he or she knows the person inside the home is baking. Learning from experience is also a form of sensible knowledge. An example is when, in class, a person learns the energy formula $KE = .5 \times m \times v^2$ from the professor. Another example is going to the library to extract the formula from one of the available books.

Knowledge gained through *understanding* is created in the mind through a thoughtful process. If we take the creation of Albert Einstein's equation for energy ($E = mc^2$), Einstein's idea actually came out of another idea: the theory of special relativity. Although there are two sources of knowledge, all our knowledge starts with the senses. From there, it proceeds to understanding.

Bibliography

1 Kahneman, D. *Thinking Fast and Slow.* 1ˢᵗ ed. New York, NY: Farrar, Strauss, and Giroux, 2011.

2 Esmaeilpour, T, Fereydouni, E., Dehghani, F., et al. "An Experimental Investigation of Ultraweak Photon Emission from Adult Murine Neural Stem Cells." *Scientific Reports* 2020; 10 (1): 463.

3 Zarkeshian, P., Kumar, S., Tuszynski, J., Barclay, P., and Simon, C. "Are there optical communication channels in the brain?" *Front Biosci (Landmark Ed)* 2018; 23: 1407–1421.

4 Folstein, J., Palmeri, T. J., Van Gulick, A. E., and Gauthier, I. "Category Learning Stretches Neural Representations in Visual Cortex." *Current Directions in Psychological Science* 2015; 24 (1): 17–23.

5 Hume, D. *A Treatise of Human Nature.* New York, NY: Penguin Books, 1740.

6 Wolfgang, L. D. *Understanding Basic Electronics.* Newington, CT: The American Radio Relay League Inc., 1992.

7 Martinez-Banaclocha, M., and Martínez Banaclocha, H. "Neuron-Astroglial Communication in Short-Term Memory: Bio-Electric, Bio-Magnetic and Bio-Photonic Signals?" 2012: 101–128.

8 Salari, V., Valian, H., Bassereh, H., Bókkon, I., and Barkhordari, A. "Ultraweak photon emission in the brain." *J Integr Neurosci* 2015; 14 (3): 419–429.

9 Shainline, J. M. "Fluxonic processing of photonic synapse events." *IEEE Journal of Selected Topics in Quantum Electronics* 2020; 26 (1): 1–15.

10 Rao-Ruiz, P., Visser, E., Mitrić, M., Smit, A. B., and van den Oever, M. C. "A Synaptic Framework for the Persistence of Memory Engrams." *Front Synaptic Neurosci* 2021; 13: 661476.

11 Ricker, T.J., Vergauwe, E., and Cowan, N. "Decay theory of immediate memory: From Brown (1958) to today (2014)." *Quarterly Journal of Experimental Psychology (2006)* 2016; 69 (10): 1969–1995.

12 Fares, R. P., Belmeguenai, A., Sanchez, P. E., et al. "Standardized environmental enrichment supports enhanced brain plasticity in healthy rats and prevents cognitive impairment in epileptic rats." *PloS One* 2013; 8 (1): e53888.

13 Jung, C. K., and Herms, J. "Structural dynamics of dendritic spines are influenced by an environmental enrichment: an in vivo imaging study." *Cerebral Cortex (New York, NY: 1991)* 2014; 24 (2): 377–384.

14 Ene, D., Der, G., Fletcher-Watson, S., et al. "Associations of Socioeconomic Deprivation and Preterm Birth With Speech, Language, and Communication Concerns Among Children Aged 27 to 30 Months." *JAMA Network Open* 2019; 2 (9): e1911027.

15 Squire, L. R. "Memory systems of the brain: a brief history and current perspective." *Neurobiology of Learning and Memory* 2004; 82 (3): 171–177.

16 McClelland, J. L., McNaughton, B. L., and O'Reilly, R. C. "Why there are complementary learning systems in the hippocampus and neocortex: insights from the successes and failures of connectionist models of learning and memory." *Psychological Review* 1995; 102 (3): 419–457.

17 Zhang, Y., and Gruber, R. "Can Slow-Wave Sleep Enhancement Improve Memory? A Review of Current Approaches and Cognitive Outcomes." *The Yale Journal of Biology and Medicine* 2019; 92 (1): 63–80.

18 Rasch, B., and Born, J. "About sleep's role in memory." *Physiological Reviews* 2013; 93 (2): 681–766.

19 Ackermann, S., and Rasch, B. "Differential effects of non-REM and REM sleep on memory consolidation?" *Current Neurology and Neuroscience Reports* 2014; 14 (2): 430.

20 Pereira de Vasconcelos, A., and Cassel, J. C. "The nonspecific thalamus: A place in a wedding bed for making memories last?" *Neuroscience and Biobehavioral Reviews* 2015; 54: 175–196.

21 Purves, D., Augustine, G. J., Fitzpatrick, D., Hall, W. C., LaMantia, A-S., and White, L. E. *Neuroscience.* 5th ed. Sunderland, MA: Sinauer Associates Inc., 2012.

22 Sherman, S. M. "Thalamus plays a central role in ongoing cortical functioning." *Nature Neuroscience* 2016; 19 (4): 533–541.

23 Bickford, M. E. "Thalamic Circuit Diversity: Modulation of the Driver/ Modulator Framework." *Frontiers in Neural Circuits* 2015; 9: 86.

24 Mitchell, A. S. "The mediodorsal thalamus as a higher order thalamic relay nucleus important for learning and decision-making." *Neuroscience and Biobehavioral Reviews* 2015; 54: 76–88.

25 Guyton, A. C., and Hall, J. E. *Textbook of Medical Physiology.* 9th ed. Philadelphia, PA: W. B. Saunders Company, 1996.

26 Sherman, S. M., and Guillery, R. W. "On the actions that one nerve cell can have on another: distinguishing 'drivers' from 'modulators.'" *Proceedings of the National Academy of Sciences of the United States of America* 1998; 95 (12): 7121–7126.

27 Bartol, T. M., Bromer, C., Kinney, J., et al. "Nanoconnectomic upper bound on the variability of synaptic plasticity." *eLife* 2015; 4: e10778.

28 Alivisatos, A. P., Chun, M., Church, G. M., Greenspan, R. J., Roukes, M. L., and Yuste, R. "The brain activity map project and the challenge of functional connectomics." *Neuron* 2012; 74 (6): 970–974.

29 Lovejoy, C. O. "The origin of man." *Science* 1981; 211 (4480): 341–350.

30 Moustafa, A. A., McMullan, R. D., Rostron, B., Hewedi, D. H., and Haladjian, H. H. "The thalamus as a relay station and gatekeeper: relevance to brain disorders. *Reviews in the Neurosciences* 2017; 28 (2): 203–218.

31 Ward, L. M. "The thalamus: gateway to the mind." *Wiley Interdisciplinary Reviews Cognitive Science* 2013; 4 (6): 609–622.

32 Fernandez de Molina y Cañas, A. "El sistema talamo-cortical y la consciencia." *Anales de la Real Academia Nacional de Medicina* 2000; 117 (4): 855–869.

33 Berger M, Garcia PS. "Anesthetic Suppression of Thalamic High-Frequency Oscillations: Evidence that the Thalamus Is More Than Just a Gateway to Consciousness?" *Anesth Analg.* 2016; 122 (6): 1737–1739.

34 Redinbaugh, M. J., Phillips, J. M., Kambi, N. A., et al. "Thalamus Modulates Consciousness via Layer-Specific Control of Cortex." *Neuron* 2020; 106 (1): 66–75.e12.

35 Glanz, K., Lewis, F. M., and Rimer, B. K. *Health Behaviors and Health Education: Theory, Research, and Practice.* 2nd ed. San Francisco, CA: Joswy-Bass Publishers, 1997.

36 Gilson, E. *The Philosophy of St. Thomas Aquinas.* New York, NY: Dorset Press, 1924.

37 Kant, I. *Critique of Pure Reason.* New York, NY: St. Martin's Press, 1929.

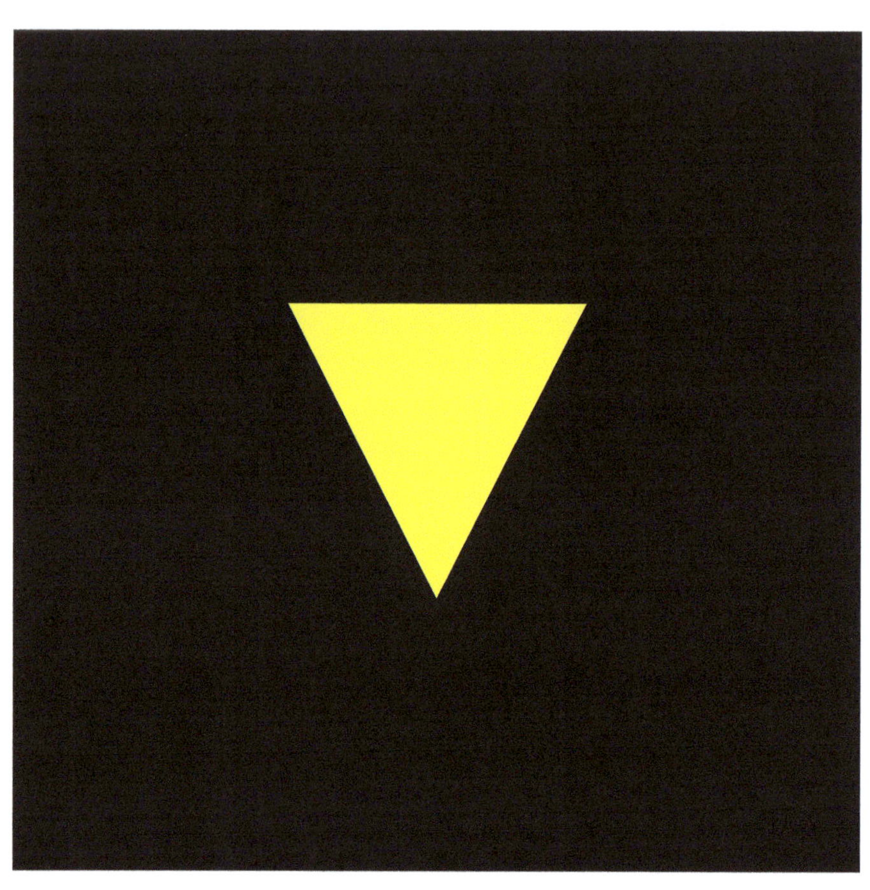

CHAPTER 3

Communicative Force
The Connection

The purpose of the communicative force is to build community. If we had no intention to connect with others or to form groups, then there would be no need for communicative force. The communicative force is powerful and can have an impact, either favorable or unfavorable, on people's attitudes, beliefs, knowledge, and behaviors. The communicative force is closely tied to the cognitive force.

The communicative force transfers energy in the form of messages from one individual or body to another. These messages are electromagnetic. This is how information or data is passed along. The bodies involved in the transfer processes are anybody and anything, and they can be animate or inanimate. A sign on the corner can inform a person to stop; a dog growling can send the message to an individual he had better cross the street (and fast!). A grimace on a person's face can inform another of that person's feelings. All these examples are forms of nonverbal communication. Communication is usually understood to mean language. But as revealed through these examples, the communicative force exchanges messages between intraspecies and interspecies. Still, in this book, I will focus mostly on language, which of course is limited to human communication.

How Communication Begins

The process begins with two bodies emitting, transmitting, and receiving ideas to get, keep, and increase the four necessities: health, status, wealth, and basic drives (see chapter 1). The *emitting* body retrieves ideas from its own brain, which encodes them into exportable messages for its motor body parts (extremities, facial muscles, or vocal cords) to transmit. The messages then are *transmitted* through space by light, sound, and smells, or through direct contact via touch and taste.

The *receiving body* then decodes the messages with its sensory organs (eyes, ears, nose, fingers, and tongue) to store them in the brain and prepare a motor response if need to. The choice to respond and what to respond depends on the impression the message leaves on the receiving body. If the message has a strong effect on the four necessities, then a motor response is more likely to be evoked. Otherwise, it is likely that just a feeling or a thought is incited.

The *transmission* is conducted through the communicative force. This force is not the emitting body, the messenger, or the receiving body alone but the relationship that develops when all three connect with one another. Something travels in between the two bodies that alter feelings, thoughts, and motor responses in both bodies. This "something" is the messengers (or transmission)—usually light and sound.

For communication to be complete, an impression (a feeling, a thought, a motor response) should be made in the receiving body. Once an impression is made, it is not necessary that there be a motor response to "close" the communication loop. Or just a feeling (happy, angry) or a thought (helpful, useless) will suffice.

Let us explore the communication loop using an example from everyday life. Let's say a person sends an email to a coworker, but the coworker never receives the email. If this is the case, then communication did not occur. However, if the individual sends an email to a coworker and the coworker reads that message, then communication occurred. Through the simple act of reading the message, the receiver is feeling and thinking. Whether the coworker then produces a motor response or not as a result of the read message is not a requirement for communication to have occurred.

Or let's say a dog shows a sign of wanting to play, but the owner does not perceive that signal; here, communication did not occur. If, however, the pet shows a sign of wanting to play and the owner perceives this signal but refuses to play, then communication did occur. The owner's choice not to play is a response.

For communication to occur, the signal sent by the emitter should alter the feelings or thoughts of the receiver. The receiver can respond with a feeling in the heart, a thought in the brain, or (hopefully not!) a punch on the nose.

Communicative contact could be intentional or incidental. Intentional transmissions are aimed at a particular body or bodies and are usually planned with the expectation of evoking a response. Incidental transmissions are unintentionally sent, and the untargeted receiver may or may not respond to them. These are impulsive in nature.

When an employee is repeatedly late to work and his supervisor writes up the employee, this is an intentional communicative contact. If, however, the employee's coworker overheard that the supervisor is going to be writing up the employee, the coworker decides that he will make sure he himself is never going to be late to work in the future is an example of incidental communicative contact. In both cases, the contact evoked a feeling, a thought, or a motor response in the receiver.

Messages

The communicative force is the process by which messages are being emitted, transmitted, and received. At the core of each message is an idea. Ideas are attitudes, beliefs, and knowledge represented in the mind as visual images. Attitudes, beliefs, and knowledge are the "voltage" that pushes the body of the emitter to transmit. You might remember from previous chapters that attitudes are feelings (likes or dislikes), beliefs are strong convictions that something is true, and knowledge is facts. A communicative message can convey any one of these three:

- Attitude: "I dislike you. Get someone else to help you" or "I like it. I will support it."
- Belief: "This cause is worthwhile. I will fight till the end" or "I don't believe we can compete with them."
- Knowledge: "The distance between home and work is three miles on the highway and two and a half miles through the streets."

Attitudes are affective and felt; beliefs and knowledge are cognitive and thoughtful. Attitudes are immediate defenders of the four necessities while beliefs and knowledge are delayed defenders. Let me explain.

Let's say a corporation's chief executive officer sends an annual report to its stockholders in which the CEO has written extensively about the company's "bright" future and also presented a financial statement showing there have been "losses." After that, she then gives a "touching" speech to the company's stockholders that cover the challenges, her positive attitude, and future directions. At the core of the CEO's transmission are the three types of messages: attitude, belief, and knowledge. Knowledge is the financial statement showing losses; belief is that the company will do well in the future; and attitude is the uplifting speech.

Humans are not born with attitudes, beliefs, and knowledge. Nor do they possess a gene for these either. Instead, attitudes, beliefs, and knowledge exist out in the socio-environment (home, school, neighborhoods, community) ready to be learned. The socio-environmental force is the instructor of attitudes, beliefs, and knowledge (to be explained in chapter 4).

The Light Bulb of Ideas

Ideas (attitudes, beliefs, and knowledge) hardly ever enter the receiving body in their pure form. When the ideas of the emitting and receiving bodies (respectively) come into contact, the contact may form new ideas. That's because the receiving body has its own ideas that serve as a filter to any incoming ideas. Incoming ideas are screened and if the receiving body allows them to enter, the ideas "amalgamate" with existing ideas. The incoming ideas then may be modified from their original form. Or an idea can just be rejected. The communicator uses one framework while the listener uses another framework to understand the message.

Let us use an example to better our understanding of the amalgamation of ideas. A medical student who just graduated from medical school was trained at a university that put emphasis on the personal rapport with and thorough physical examination of the patient to make a diagnosis. This medical student has preset ideas that favor the interview, physical examination, and the personal touch. The same medical student then enters a residency program that undermines the humane interaction and puts more weight on the use of modern technology to make a diagnosis. As the second mode of medical practice filters through the mind of the medical student, his or her ideas change to value both, the human touch complemented by medical technology.

Mediums for Transmission

The medium for the transmission of messages is quite important, and it can vary from message to message. Returning to the earlier example, the CEO who wrote the annual report is the emitter; light and sound are the transmitters of the CEO's messages, and the stockholders are the receivers. Specifically, the CEO emits by writing and talking, and the stockholders receive by reading and hearing. When the stockholders open up the annual report and view the actual pages, it is light waves traveling from the print to the retina that allows them to view the pages; when the CEO makes her speech, it is sound waves traveling from the mouth to the ears.[1] The CEO and stockholders communicate by light waves (writing) and sound waves (speech) but hopefully not by touch (pushing)!

The communicative force consists of both verbal and nonverbal communication. Many nonverbal communications—postures, gestures, and grimaces, for example—can be emitted simultaneously with communications that utilize language. Many times, these verbal and nonverbal communications give off mixed signals. Continuing with our current example, when the CEO is being questioned by stockholders, she may communicate positive verbal messages but show facial signs of her displeasure at being questioned, such as pursed lips.

The use of words can be ambiguous, as people often speak in figurative language, either indirectly or unintentionally. So a complete breakdown of communication can occur if the encoded message differs from the decoded message.

Let's say a driver stops at a stop sign and asks his passenger if anything is coming from his side of the street. The passenger responds, "A dog." So the driver seeing that the dog is not in front decides to proceed. Well, the car's passage is stopped when suddenly a Greyhound (the passenger's "dog") bus strikes the car! This example illustrates the adverse effects that can occur with a breakdown in communication.

Communication Modes

Communicators can be a cell, a plant, an ant, an elephant, or a human, as nonhumans and humans frequently communicate with each other. For example, when a person waters a plant, the plant receives the message of nourishment; when a person turns on the kitchen light, a roach in his kitchen receives the message to take cover; and when ants bite a person, it sends a message to that person to get out of their territory! All these occur because (as explained in the previous chapter) when the amygdala-thalamus-cerebral cortex deliberate, and a decision is made. They then send a command to the muscular system.

When we apply this understanding to the communicative force, the motor cortex responses are calls, displays, vocalizations, drawings, speech, and writing. A *call* is an utterance, a *display* is a bodily expression, a *vocalization* is a sound, a *drawing* is an illustration, *speech* is the use of spoken phrases, and *writing* is the use of written phrases.

Calls, vocalizations, and speech are sound-based; displays, drawings, and writings are light-based. Calls, displays, vocalizations, and drawings are nonlanguage; speech and writing are language. Nonlanguage communication emits mostly attitudes; and language communication emits attitudes, beliefs, and/or knowledge. All are communicative forces.

How the Modes of Communication Developed

Calls, displays, vocalizations, drawings, speech, and writing appear in the same order throughout child development as they did in human evolution. In order of appearance, first came calls and displays, second came vocalizations and drawings, and third came speech and writing.

Since child development is a better-understood science today, the following are some approximate time frames as to when the communication modes universally appear.[2, 3]

In Childhood

First on the scene are calls and displays. Newborns release a fretful cry to communicate that they are hungry or in pain, and they release a sigh when their hunger or pain has been relieved. At four months of age, infants display a social smile to communicate acceptance; at six months, they display facial expressions of anger to communicate being upset; and at eleven months they gesture with their hands and arms to communicate that they want something. Such early forms of communication are universal. A Chinese, Syrian, and German child crying will all be doing so to communicate the same meaning: one of displeasure.

The next modes of communication to appear in child development are vocalizations and drawings. Infants vocalize their first word around the age of twelve months and scribble their first drawing around the age of eighteen months. Infants usually use vocals and drawings to communicate their most basic wants—for example, to call for their parents, to ask for food, and to relieve their discomfort.

The last modes of communication to appear are speech and writing. Generally, a child at the age of six years will form a complex speech pattern and, at the age of nine years, write in complete sentences.

In Human Evolution

When it comes to human evolution, the modes of communication appeared in the same sequence as in childhood development. Specifically, calls and displays are the earliest forms of communication in human evolution and could have appeared as early as four million years ago with *Australopithecus afarensis.*[4] Early humans probably had certain cries and laughter to express discomfort and pleasure. Scientists think they may have had forty to fifty different calls to communicate with each other and that their messages were likely to be about food, sex, and predators. Similarly, showing the canine teeth was a display of anger, and dancing was a display of joy.

These assumptions scientists have made about early humans are based on hominid predecessors, as primates have thirty to forty calls to communicate with each other. For example, monkeys have a "booming" call that alerts other monkeys when a food tree is discovered. Young monkeys call out in a distinctive way to their parents when they are hungry. Vervet monkeys have one call if a ground predator (snake) approaches and another call if a sky predator (hawk) approaches. The ground predator call warns other monkeys to climb up a tree, and the sky predator call alerts other monkeys to run down to the ground.

Vocalizations and drawings were the second set of communicative forces to develop. Other than the upright position, another distinguishing feature that separated humans from nonhumans was vocalizations. Vocalization is the pronunciation of a word. The first vocalizations were probably onomatopoetic (words associated with the sound they imitate, phonetic). For example, to describe a bear, early humans might have uttered *grrrwal*; to describe a buffalo, they might have used *moo*; and to describe a cat, they might have vocalized *meow*.

Vocalizations may have evolved around 2.5 million years ago in the *Homo habilis.*[5] *Homo habilis* was the human ancestor to boast the most significant increase in brain size. From *Australopithecus* to *Homo habilis* the brain size increased by 50 percent, from Homo habilis to *Homo erectus* it increased by 25 percent, and from *Homo erectus* to present-day *Homo sapiens* it increased by 35 percent. A second feature different in *Homo habilis* from its predecessor hominid was the descent of the vocal tracts, something important for vocal range and flexibility in terms of sound production. The third feature that stood out in *Homo habilis* was the ability to use hand-held stone tools to cut flesh and chop bones. The first chopped-up bones appear in fossil records around 2.5 million years ago. This evolution of the brain, vocal cords, and hands in *Homo habilis* were three anatomical changes necessary for vocal articulation and physical manipulation.

Just like it did with vocalizations, *Homo habilis* used drawings to communicate mental representations of real items or events in their universe. The oldest cave drawing, discovered at Pettakere Cave in Sulawesi, Indonesia, is thirty-five thousand years old and depicts human hands and animals.[6] The first drawings were pictograms. *Pictograms* are drawings associated with a mental image that, in turn, represented a particular object or event in the universe. For example, a drawing of a buffalo was associated with a mental image of a buffalo, and a drawing of a spear was associated with a mental image of a spear. By combining several pictograms, *Homo habilis* could form and communicate ideas. For example, the drawings of a buffalo and a spear together were associated with the idea, "Let's go and hunt buffalos for food and clothes." The drawings of buffalo and spear together formed what is called an *ideogram,* a written symbol that indicates the idea of a thing but that lacks the sounds to say it.

The last communication modes to appear are speech and writing, which are the origins of language. The Sumerian civilization created these around five thousand years ago in Mesopotamia (present day Iraq).[7] Speech and writing allow the mind to fancy and imagine things. Imagination grabs all associations and combines them to form new and more elaborate forms of speaking and writing. Imagination is an operant form of thinking. It can transpose and change. It brings consequences into the decision-making process. And it sets up the question, "What if?"

In the truest sense of the word, language came into existence once an agreed-upon set of symbols were coded to be associated with particular sounds. The association of symbols or letters with sounds would become the root of all languages and the basic building blocks of the alphabet. The socio-environmental force is the originator of the coded symbols. More on this in chapter 4.

The Phoenicians, who lived three thousand years ago, were the first to create an alphabet.[7] The Phoenicians lived along the Mediterranean in present-day Lebanon. The Phoenicians then spread across Greece, Italy, North Africa, and Spain, taking with them their alphabet. This alphabet would be the roots of the Aramaic (Old Testament language), the Arab, and the Hebrew alphabets.

The Greeks living 2,500 years ago adopted the Phoenician alphabet and modified it to fit into their own language. The Greeks were the first to introduce vowels into the alphabet. The Greek alphabet had twenty-four letters (seventeen consonants and seven vowels). It was the source of the Latin alphabet (2,300 years ago), and the Latin alphabet is what is currently used in the English language.

The Modes Mingle

Although the forms of communication evolved at different stages, the more modern ones never replaced the primitive ones. Instead, they coexist. Present-day humans sometimes use calls, displays, vocals, pictures, speech, and writing— all in one communicative response.

However, the different forms of expressions in one emission sometimes are in agreement while at other times they are in disagreement. When insulted, a person might emit a call of doubt ("hmm"), a display of displeasure (facial grimace), and a speech of reconciliation ("let's work it out") all in one instant.

Many times, our language communications (beliefs and knowledge) will keep our nonlanguage communications (attitudes) in check. Yet many times, nonlanguage communications leave a greater impression on us than language communications!

Tables 1 to 4 demonstrate examples of modern calls and displays. The examples in these tables demonstrate calls and displays with their corresponding message.

Table 1. Calls	
Calls	Attitude emitted
Ouch!	"I dislike the situation. I am in pain."
Oh!	"I dislike the situation. I am disappointed."
Yeah!	"I like the situation. I am happy"
Wow!	"I like the situation. I am impressed."
Hey!	"I dislike you. I disagree with what you did."
Voice Tone	
Harsh	"I dislike the situation. I will make my point."
Soft	"I like you. I respect you."

Table 2. Displays (facial)	
Expression	Attitude Emitted
Wrinkling of forehead	"I dislike you. I do not like what you are saying."
Single eye wink	"I like you. You are attractive."
Puckered eyes	"I dislike you. I do not trust you."
Puckered lips	"I like you. I am sending you a kiss."
Smile	"I like you. You are nice."
Tongue stuck out	"I dislike you. You are not nice."
Dropped lower jaw and mouth agape	"I dislike you. I cannot believe what you did."
Lips shut tight and corners pulling down	"I dislike you. I am upset."

Table 3. Displays (arm and hand)	
Posture	Attitude Emitted
Palm of hand in the "stop" position	"I dislike you. Do not get close."
Hand to lip than blowing air off palm	"I like you. I am sending you a kiss."
Arms crossed	"I dislike this. I am not interested."
Index and middle finger in a "V" shape	"I like you. Peace."
Middle finger sticking up	"I dislike you. I'm angry."
Thumbs up	"I like you. Good job."
Gesture	
A hug	"I like you. You are nice."
Curling index finger back and forth	"I like you. Come here."
Turning index finger from side to side	"I dislike your action. Do not do it again."
Covered mouth with hand	"I dislike what I said. I am sorry."

Table 4. Displays (legs and trunk)	
Posture	Attitude Emitted
Slouching in chair	"I dislike the situation. I am bored."
One leg in front and chest pushed forward	"I dislike the situation. I will challenge it."
Feet place opposite direction of speaker	"I dislike you. I am not interested."
Gesture	
Kicked the ground	"I dislike the situation. I am upset."

Walked away from speaker	"I dislike you. I am not taking your nuance."
Ran away from the attacker	"I dislike you. I am scared."
Dancing	"I like this; this is fun."

Gene or Culture?

Now that we understand a bit about how language developed in humans, this understanding begs a question: *How did humans acquire language?* There is no agreement among scientists on this question. One group claims that it was genes while the other claims culture.

An Argument for Genes

In terms of the gene group, they argue that there is a specific gene in the DNA and a specific center in the brain that turns "on" to initiate language in children. This mechanism (also called *universal grammar*) consists of an innate device that automatically turns on speech in children without effort or formal instruction.[4, 8] According to this method, the brain comes "preprogrammed" with a mechanism that can build an unlimited set of sentences out of a finite list of words. Here is an analogy that can be used to explain this mechanism: Infants are born with complex audio equipment that has unlabeled knobs and switches, and they also are missing the instructional manual. But by listening to their own calls and vocalizations, infants can begin creating their instructional manual. Because the capacity for language has not changed in the last eighty thousand years, the gene group claims that language emerged suddenly after a gene mutation. They consider language a Darwinian evolutionary adaptation, just like hand dexterity and blue eyes are.

To have one gene mutation ignite language is a big feat. First, for language to emerge, it needed the coordination of five speech organs (larynx, epiglottis, soft palate, tongue, and lips), nearly one hundred muscles, and the enlarged cerebral cortex to fall into perfect anatomical position and physiology for speech to occur.[9]

Second, the problem with the gene theory is that a specific gene and a specific brain organ for language have not been found. Moreover, language did not appear suddenly; it took at least four million years to evolve! Additionally, it did not begin as language. It began as primitive calls and vocalizations, and from these, it evolved into language. It is my opinion, therefore, that the idea of a gene suddenly occurring to "turn on" language overnight is hard to accept. A multitude of mutations to a bunch of genes would have been needed to instruct speech organs and the brain to handle language.

An Argument for Culture

The communicative force is inseparable from the cognitive force; language and brain evolved beside one another. Both evolved through the acquisition of knowledge and skills through experience and study. Humans were not born with knowledge and skills; they acquired them from the social environment. Learning occurred in a particular context (home, school, library, work) by using sense (eyes, ears) and motor organs (epiglottis, hands) to input and operate the learned material. Language thus was learned within a rich and elaborate social context.[5]

Language is a social product. Children who grow up in the wild demonstrate considerable difficulty learning a new language and exhibit permanent language deficits. Furthermore, children raised by educated parents develop a richer and more elaborate language than children raised by less educated parents.[10] Children growing up in disadvantaged households have a six-month gap in language development compared with children growing up in more advantaged households. Other scientists have also shown the strong influence that the social environment has on language.[11, 12]

Language is a constituent of culture, and culture is a product of society. Culture consists of many components (religion, food, technology, education, socioeconomic status), but of all of them, language is the most significant.

Culture, like genes, can be transmitted from one generation to the next, like the culture of poverty.[13] Similarly, toolmaking was a cultural revolution 2.5 million years ago. It did not originate from a gene mutation. It was a skill learned in one generation and passed on to the next generation.

Parts of culture are beliefs and knowledge. The ability to believe in something is what changed the brain structures that support language. Once humans were endowed with the ability to believe, their expectations changed. Through believing, humans had hope. They could hope for better ways to live longer; develop relationships; and clothe, shelter, and transport. Knowledge allowed humans to measure antecedents to assess consequents. Believing allowed humans to consider the impossible when considering options to get, keep, and increase the four necessities. The capacity for knowledge and beliefs allowed humans to remember their histories and explore their futures.

But beliefs and knowledge were only thoughts; to become operational, they needed an instrument. That instrument was language. Humans needed to develop language and the structures that support it to realize their beliefs.

The hypothesis in this book thus is that language did not only enter a person from the outside; it was self-actualized in humans by the socio-environmental force and stationed in the cerebral cortex to use. And when done, it goes back to the socio-environmental force.[5] Like the case with a library book, language does not belong to the individual; it is borrowed.

From the perspective of culture, it was language that shaped the cerebral cortex and not that the cerebral cortex shaped language.

Cerebral Cortex

The cerebral cortex is the brain processing center of the communicative force. The cerebral cortex consists of two hemispheres (a right and a left) and four lobes (the temporal, frontal, parietal, and occipital) (see figure 1). (Note: there is a fifth lobe, which will be explained in chapter 4.) The left hemisphere is the dominant side for language, yet without the right hemisphere, a long conversation cannot be sustained. Both hemispheres thus play essential and complementary roles.

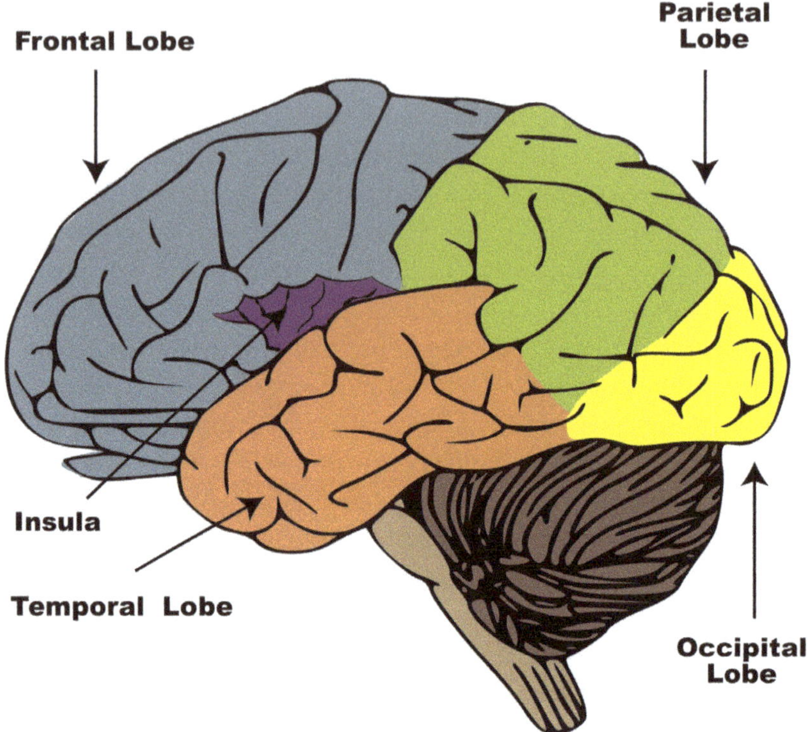

Figure 1. Four lobes and insular cortex

In this section, I will discuss the communicative force with a focus on language. Language encompasses hearing, reading, spelling, speaking, writing, drawing, and math. The classic model of language originated in the nineteenth century.[14] According to this theory, language was localized to two brain areas: the left temporal and frontal lobes. The temporal lobe was responsible for *decoding* (reception of) language and the frontal lobe for *encoding* (production of) language.

With the advent of modern technology, particularly neuroimaging and electrical brain mapping, new knowledge about the anatomy and physiology of language was learned. The new knowledge showed that brain highways, instead of brain areas, better explained the operation of language.[15, 16] These information superhighways, called fasciculi, operate like fiber optic bundles through which the communicative force is conducted across the four lobes.

The communicative force conducted along the fasciculus or white matter tracts comes in different intensities and complexities. If the communicative force is unintelligible, then the message does not go further than the temporal lobe.[17] But if it is intelligible, then the temporal lobe (primary auditory cortex), as the port of entry, channels it to one or more of the other three lobes.

If the temporal lobe channels the message, the most likely next stop for that message is the frontal lobe. In fact, the communication tracts between the temporal and frontal lobes are more numerous than those between any of the other lobes.

The frontal lobe has two physiological distinct areas: the prefrontal cortex and the motor cortex. The prefrontal cortex handles language planning, and the motor cortex produces language execution. The prefrontal lobe handles the more complex messages coming from the socio-environmental force (via the insular cortex, see chapter 4) or those mentally evoked.[18, 19] Its primary role is understanding, and its secondary role is planning. Planning involves the executive control of language production in the form of verbal or written strategies.

Although the primary role of the prefrontal lobe is to understand, when it comes to more in-depth comprehension and specialization, the temporal and prefrontal lobes recruit the parietal and occipital lobes, as well as the two hemispheres. The temporal-occipital juncture forms the visual word form area or VWFA.[20] The VWFA is a specialized area associated with reading (silent and out loud), spelling, and writing.

The VWFA is active in literate (and not illiterate) adults.[21] Blind people who learn Braille have an active VWFA. Such findings indicate that the literacy skill did not come "from the factory" but is learned "on the road," so to speak.

The drawing of objects and geometric shapes activates the frontal-parietal juncture.[22] These make sense, as drawing is just as, or even more, complex than handwriting. Drawing involves motor activity, creativeness, and placement in space. Handwriting involves only one brain hemisphere while drawing involves both.

The frontal-parietal juncture is also involved with math problems.[23] These lobes are sensitive to addition, multiplication, and changes in the cardinality of a set of objects. Like word complexity, prefrontal activation increases as the complexity of the math problem increases. And similar to drawing, the representation of numbers activates both brain hemispheres.[20]

Once the four cerebral cortex lobes have processed language and a response is ready to be delivered, it is the frontal motor cortex that pulls the lever. The motor cortex has strong innervation to all the muscles involved with speech, and to the arms and hands if the response is written. In fact, many times speech is accompanied by a hand display, like in the case when someone cuts in front of a person who is driving, and that person responds with an angry flailing of the hand and a strongly worded yell.

If the motor cortex executes the same performance repetitively, that performance becomes a skill. Skill learning is the sum of attitudes, beliefs, and knowledge. Yet not all skills are desirable. Literary and manual labor skills are, while hacking and identity theft are not.

With the cognitive force, the thalamus is the main driver; but with the communicative force, the thalamus oversight lessens. The thalamus continues to focus on heightened attention, memory, and relaying language inputs (read and heard) up to the cerebral cortex. Once information is inside the cortex, the creation, processing, and production of language is a matter of the cerebral cortex and the socio-environmental force.

We know the role of the thalamus lessens as lesions to the thalamus have produced mild language deficits, which include semantic substitutions and the repetition of complex utterances.[16, 24, 25] Speech, however, remains intact; and the language deficits last at most a week with most afflicted individuals recovering completely.

The socio-environmental force is of paramount importance when it comes to language. Society creates rules and principles that govern language by means of an agreed-upon convention. These prescriptive rules dictate to the speaker and writer the way accepted modes of language should be spoken and written, respectively. This social convention developed a menu of terms by which language abides (see table 5). This terminology is too specialized for the thalamus to have handled alone and for a gene to have mutated.

Table 5. List of terms that govern language	
Phonetics	Speech sounds
Lexicon	List of words
Semantics	Linguistic meaning
Morphemes	Building blocks that make up a word
Syntax	Structure of sentences
Grammar	Set of rules governing the correct use of language
Prosody	Patterns of rhythm, stress, and intonation in a language
Orthographic	Rules of spelling, hyphenation, capitalization, word breaks, emphasis, and punctuation
Grapheme	Smallest unit of writing, which includes alphabetic letters, typographic ligatures, Chinese characters, numerical digits, punctuation marks, and other individual symbols
Phoneme	Units of sound that distinguish one word from another—for example, *p*, *b*, *d*, and *t* in the English words *pad*, *pat*, *bad*, and *bat*
Concepts	Grouping things that are similar in some respect into classes

What's New?

This is preliminary research, but it is worth mentioning before leaving this section. New studies are suggesting that the insular cortex, or insula, plays an important role in language, similar to what the thalamus is to the cognitive force.[15, 26] The insula is located between the temporal and frontal lobes. If both lobes are separated, it is possible to see the insula (see figure 1).

The reason the insula is being suggested as a language nexus is because of the strong connections it has with the temporal (reception) and frontal (production) lobes. In addition, the insula participates in brain circuits that relay language information to the other cerebral lobes, initiates and maintains language, and is vital when needing to learn new aspects of speech. The insula thus appears to be a core area in language reception, processing, and production. More about the insula in chapter 4.

Sense Organs

The socio-environmental force creates language, and language is introduced to the individual by means of the sense organs. The sense organs are the skin, nose, tongue, ears, and eyes. The role of sense organs is to function as transducers. They translate the input energy of one form into the output energy of another form.

Sense organs capture language through hair follicles.[1] Yes, hairs! Hairs are the microscopic receptors on the skin, nose, tongue, ears, and eyes.

Skin hairs are the first to detect movement or pressure. Any slight movement of skin hairs stimulates the nerve fibers entwining the root of the hair. Taste buds consist of tiny hairs embedded on the tongue's surface. These tiny hairs detect the four qualities of taste: bitter, sour, sweet, and salty. (Humans favor salty and sweet and avoid bitter and sour tastes.) Tiny hairs on the surface of the nose detect odor. There are perhaps one hundred primary odors that nasal hairs can detect. Hairs inside the ear detect vibrations of air pressure waves. Hairs (cones and rods) are photoreceptors located in the retina that detect light waves.

When any of the aforementioned hairs are brushed by mechanical, chemical, and electromagnetic stimuli, it activates the respective sense organs. On the receiving end, the receptors in the sense organs are mechanoreceptors, chemoreceptors, and electromagnetoreceptors.

The skin and ears are mechanoreceptors. *Mechanoreceptors* are hairs that detect mechanical deformations by direct physical contact or by air vibrations exerting pressure on the receptors. The nose and tongue are chemoreceptors. *Chemoreceptors* are hairs that detect chemical substances (odors, fragrances) by direct contact applied to the receptors. The eyes are electromagnetoreceptors. *Electromagnetoreceptors* are hairs that detect photons striking electrons on the receptor. The ears also can detect electromagnetic waves. Television and radio waves are a type of electromagnetic energy that travels without the need for a medium. Sound waves, in turn, need a medium such as air conduction to travel.

Hairs on the skin, tongue, ears, and eyes uptake external stimuli and direct them to the thalamus for sorting and modulating. From the thalamus, the messages are passed on to the cerebral cortex for processing.

Hairs from the nose are the only receptors not to direct their messages to the thalamus; instead, they direct their messages to the amygdala. Why? Well, odors are exclusively sensual. The smell of food or the smell of perfume may stir passion without a thought.

All the sense organs can receive the socio-environmental force. A rich fragrance on a date, a tasteful chocolate for valentines, and a slap to the face—all can communicate a message. For the purpose of language, though, it is eye and ear hairs that matter.

Our Language Messengers

Eye and ear hairs receive messages carried by the messengers of light and sound through space and time. The space between encoding (emitting) a message and decoding (receiving) a message is either a vacuum or medium. Light waves travel through a *vacuum* (electromagnetic field) and sound waves through a *medium* (air). Radio waves are a type of electromagnetic radiation.

The time or speed of light and sound is measured in miles (or kilometers) per hour. The speed of a sound leaving a person's mouth toward an individual's ears is approximately 761 mph. The speed of a photon (a tiny light particle that moves in waves) leaving the letters of a document toward the retina is approximately 670,600,000 mph. Radio waves also travel at the speed of light. Light and radio waves are the fastest messengers, and sound waves are the next fastest.

Because of their affinity for speed, humans are mostly audiovisual. This section, therefore, will focus on the messengers of light and sound. The messages transmitted by light and sound make an impression based on their validity, clarity, and frequency. *Validity* measures intellectual complexity; it is knowledge-based. Messages based on evidence make a greater impression than those based on opinion.

Clarity measures how well the subject of the communication is articulated and reported; in this case, it is grammar. An important message with supportive evidence may not make an impression if it is not articulated properly or reported well.

Frequency measures the number of messages transmitted over a time period; it is the rate of delivery. The messaging frequency deemed effective in the world of advertising is estimated to be between ten and twenty-over months to a year.[27, 28]

Thus, a validated message that is articulated and reported still may not make much of an impression if there is a low frequency. The most impressive messages are those that are valid, clear, and repeated over time.

Light Waves

Light is the messenger for displays, drawings, and writings. When a person releases a display, a drawing, or a written message, he/she does it to send a message to an observer. The message someone is sending may be an attitude, belief, or knowledge; but in all these cases, the messenger is that of a photon.

At the time of observation, photons bounce off the gestures, drawings, or letters being released by the person. At the time of the bounce, photons pick up messages and carry them back to the retina of the observer. The photon then comes into existence as an image in the retina and brain.

The retina is not the source of photons; rather, it is the detector of photons. The sources of photons are hot bodies—things like light bulbs, fires, or the sun. These hot bodies radiate photons into the universe where they travel at the speed of light. In their travels, they illuminate objects by bouncing off their surfaces. Photons can also be absorbed or go right through the object, but for the purpose of transmitting messages, it is the bounce that picks up messages and makes them available to interested observers.

If the observer is not interested, the field of the universe remains a blur of senseless photon waves traveling in all directions and bouncing off all objects. But if the observer is interested, the act of observing freezes what are blurry photon waves into vivid visual particles.

Interestingly, what the individual chooses to observe instantly becomes his or her reality. Reality is a matter of choice. Humans are creators of their own reality, as well as victims of their own creation.

An example is a person traveling in a plane and looking down at the city below as the plane is landing. The sun sends photon waves bouncing off all the objects in the city; but the observer, in a bit of a daze thinking about work, just sees a blur of buildings, trees, sidewalks, streets, and other large objects. Within this "blur" are any one or two or more of a million realities from which the individual can choose to notice.

In this case, as the plane starts to descend and get closer to the ground below, the person observes a dilapidated apartment building. This is when the individual collapses and sees that there are children playing outdoors at a site that is filthy and in poor condition. This image may put the observer in a somber mood. So regardless of the actual situation taking place down below, the observer suddenly becomes a victim of his own creation. Many times, humans experience the universe through the narrow kaleidoscope of personal experience because they choose to experience it that way.

Extraordinary Spirits

Photons are ideal messengers because of their extraordinary characteristics. First, because photons travel at the speed of light, they are spread out across space. A photon travels so fast that it leaves a flash between two objects!

The flash of a photon is itself a string in a particular vibrational pattern. A photon traveling between the sun and earth leaves a flash of light that connects both sun and earth into one frame in space. Thus, the same photon can be on the sun, on the earth, or on both at the same time.

If an observer in space looks toward the sun, the photon will appear there; if the observer looks toward the earth, the photon will appear there. In either case, it bounces off the sun or the earth and into the retina of the observer. The photon, by some unexplained sense, "knows" where the observer will look and appears right in front of the observer's eyesight. This produces an apparition: a ghost.

What do I mean by "ghost" in this sense? Photons are the smallest constituent of the electromagnetic field. Because photons are so tiny, they are weightless, and if weightless, they are nonmaterial. And if they are nonmaterial, they must just be spirits. Next, at the speed of light, time comes to a halt. For a photon, the past, present, and future are connected by a web of radiation that sees everything at once. For photons, the beginning and the present are a one-time frame, and photons see the future too!

How? Let's take an example that is far-fetched, but the speeds quoted are actual. Let's assume a man with a gun is hiding in a dark alley waiting to shoot a woman walking by. Suddenly the man pops out and, from a block away, shoots a bullet that travels at 1,700 mph to strike the woman. Now let's also assume that at the corner of the alley is a streetlight that sends a photon to the female warning her of the approaching bullet. The bullet is traveling at 1,700 mph, and the photon is traveling at 670,600,000 mph. The photon gets there first and warns the woman ahead of time to duck! The photon went past the present and into the future (and saved the woman's life!).

Another extraordinary fact: Photons live eternally. Because photons are nonmaterial, they are not brought into life by birth and are not removed from life by death. Photons just exist.

Photons carry energy, and it is only this energy that transmutes. The energy that photons carry in the communicative force comes in the forms of attitudes, beliefs, and knowledge. It is the energy delivered in the form of attitudes, beliefs, and knowledge that evoke a person to act or react; and it can exert so much force that it can produce a bomb able to obliterate a whole city or produce an antiviral able to eradicate HIV.

If a person shows a facial expression of dislike, it is the energy inherent in the attitude that propels the targeted individual to react by walking away. If a person strongly believes that he or she can climb a mountain, then it is the energy inherent in this belief that propels the prospective climber to attempt to reach the top of the mountain.

Likewise, a scientist on a mission to find the cure for breast cancer starts with a set of knowledge. During the scientist's investigations and review of the literature, his or her initial knowledge goes through several transmutations until a final knowledge is formulated that has the potential for developing a new drug to cure breast cancer. Thus, latent energy lies in attitudes, beliefs, and knowledge; and the messenger of this energy is the photon.

It is amazing what spirits can do!

Sound Waves

Sound is the messenger for calls, vocalizations, and speech messages. With calls, vocalizations, and speech, air molecules are set in motion by sound vibrations that are produced by the vocal cords. If a person covers his mouth with his hand and makes a sound, vibrations will be felt on the hand. These sound vibrations leave the vocal cords and travel through space (and time) by pushing air molecules against each other. An air molecule travels only a short distance, but if air molecules push one another, they then can transmit the message over several hundred meters. As they travel, air molecules move closer together (condense) and then move farther apart (rarify) to produce a mechanical force. This "clump and bump" produces a pump effect that transmits the message over a long distance.

Sound energy travels in *waves*, which have three characteristics: amplitude, timbre, and frequency. *Amplitude* measures intensity, *timbre* measures sound quality, and *frequency* measures pitch. Intensity is measured in decibels and is a function of the degree to which the waves deflect upward (positive) or downward (negative). The higher the decibel, the louder the sound; and the larger the deflection, the greater the impression. A ticking watch creates a sound level of 20 decibels, and a rock concert creates a sound level of 130 decibels. Humans can hear amplitudes between twenty and sixteen thousand hertz. Any more or any less, and the human ear cannot sense it.

Timbre provides information about the quality of sound, specifically the purity or complexity of each sound wave. Thus, a violin and a drum have different timbres. Frequency measures the speed or number of wave cycles per second. So a parent reminding a child to pick up her room once a day may make a greater impression than reminding her to pick up her room once a week.

Humans can hear frequencies between twenty and twenty thousand cycles per second. If the frequencies are any less or any more than that range, humans do not have the capability of sensing the sound even though the sound is out there.

Verisimilitude

The communicative force is imprecise. There is the socio-environmental force out there with all its objects producing events. The events are encoded into messages, transmitted, and decoded at the receiving end. Yet the communication between the emitting and receiving objects is not perfect. A person sitting in an office at work is surrounded by a multitude of events that take his/her attention and hence the message may never excite his receptors. It is likely that in the background there is a copier running, a coworker talking, a fan blowing, a paperclip falling, a clock ticking, and a supervisor breaking a pencil. Each of these events is strong enough to be seen and heard by the employee, yet these are imperceptible to him.

At the macroscopic (visible to the naked eye) level, there is a copier, a coworker, a fan, a paperclip, a clock, a supervisor, and a pencil out there emitting signals, all with the potential of inciting the individual. But because the employee is focused on writing a sales strategy that will give him a raise (wealth, a necessity), all the other external events are fuzzy (sound and light) waves.

At the microscopic level, the objects surrounding the individual are a cloud of atoms oscillating back and forth.[29] Take, for example, the fingers of the supervisor breaking the pencil. Below the skin are bone and muscles, below these are tissues, below these are cells, below these are molecules, and below these are atoms oscillating back and forth. Then the pencil splits. There are wood and lead, and if that material is split again, there are wood and lead subparticles. If split again, there are wood and lead molecules; and if there is continued splitting, eventually there will remain atoms oscillating back and forth. Atoms have electrons rotating around them going so fast that they form a cloud. At the point of contact, the finger and pencil lose their borders and become an indistinct cloud of electrons. Similarly, the copier, coworker, fan, paperclip, desk, clock, supervisor, pencil, and employee have no fine borders among them. Instead, they are all interconnected forming a singularity.

A Singular Unbroken Oneness

Out there in the socio-environment is an unbroken oneness where all objects are interrelated and interacting. What affects one affects the other. If some business owners do not pay their employees enough and charge too much for the company's products, there will not be enough customers out there to afford the business owners' products. Because the owners of the business will not make enough in sales, they may have to close their stores. What goes around comes around.

What are out there are clouds of objects producing infinite events spreading throughout space and time in a fuzzy wave affecting one and all together. If what is out there is cloudy and fuzzy, then it cannot be real. But if it still has an effect, it must be *nearly* real. Nearly real means that it is subreal. Subreality, then, is what really exists out there. If the universe is surreal, how does the individual make sense of it? By observing it!

To observe is to be aware of objects and events using sense organs. When a person has an observation, waves of chemicals, odors, sounds, and lights freeze and become solid particles. Momentum halts, and the person frames the position that has formed; this position then becomes a memory. The person is the frame of reference, and from there, he or she perceives the chaotic universe.

Observing for Necessity's Sake

It is important to be aware that a person does not make an observation just for the sake of making it. An individual makes an observation because an approaching event may affect his or her four necessities. There could be a hundred—a thousand—events out there, but if they do not affect the individual's four necessities, then they remain fuzzy or blurry waves. But if they do affect those necessities, then they will demand the person's undivided attention.

Let's return to the earlier example above where the individual is working on his sales strategy. If the ceiling fan starts to fall on his head, then he will refocus his attention from the sales strategy to the ceiling fan (health). If the supervisor breaks the pencil because she is upset at the individual's performance, then the individual will refocus the attention on the boss (wealth) over concern that he or she will lose his job. If a coworker is talking negatively about the colleague, then the focus will be on the coworker's gossip (status). Because the ceiling fan, the supervisor, and the coworker suddenly threaten a necessity, these become the center of attention.

Once the individual freezes the frame, and the message is received, what the individual truly receives is an approximation of the truth or *verisimilitude*. Consider again the ceiling fan, the supervisor, and the coworker appearing to affect the individual in our example. The emission from these three objects appears real and the reception within the individual appears true, but appearances can be deceptive. The ceiling fan may have detached but still hangs on or dangles via the cord (so it was never going to hit him), the supervisor may have been in a bad mood simply because his wife was in a car accident that morning (the employee's job was never at risk), and the coworker actually was speaking disparagingly about someone else (the friendship with the individual was never in jeopardy). What the individual thought was true events were instead not real.

It's an Inexact "Science"

Another example of the inexactitude of messages is when the same event is interpreted differently by two individuals. In our example, the event is a hailstorm, and the two persons are a homeowner and an insurance agent arguing about what caused the roof damage. The homeowner attributes the roof damage to the hailstorm and the insurance agent blames preexisting conditions. The homeowner wants to get paid and the insurance agent does not want to pay, and it is all about the same event.

Another example is a foul in basketball that occurs right in front of the referee and coach. One shouts "Foul!" and the other declares stridently "No foul!" What is happening is that each individual interprets the same event from their own frame of reference.

Why is it that the individual cannot ever know the full truth of objects and events in the socio-environment? Because what the individual receives and stores in the mind is a representation of external objects and events and not the objects and events themselves. Because objects are never fully grasped, their true essence will never be known. At best, a person's sense organs construct images of objects and events and then assimilate them to accommodate the person's own set of attitudes, beliefs, and knowledge. Sense perceptions never receive objects and events in their pure form. Perceptions, therefore, are constructive.

If a bigot sees a person of color, an image and a belief will be constructed in the bigot's brain of that person. The image is a representation of that person, and the belief is that the person is inferior to those of his kind. The true essence may be that the person is not even a person of color (just appears to be) and that the person is of outstanding character and morals. Because perceptions are simply reconstructive models of the truth, they are illusory interpretations.

The Scientific Method

The purpose of science is to approximate truth or verisimilitude. We already explained that many, if not most, of the things one hears and reads are not true. Well, the scientific method is the best approach to approximate the truth. The scientific method is a rigorous and systematic approach to gaining and expanding knowledge. The scientific method is purely a linguistic process, particularly the written form. The universal language used in the scientific method is math. It is through measurement that knowledge is gained and expanded.

The scientific method starts with a problem. The problem could be complex (like determining which is a better medicine to control high blood pressure) or simple (like finding the shortest distance between home and work). The study to conduct to approximate the truth could be elaborate (like conducting an experiment with two groups [green pill vs. blue pill]) or simple (like measuring the distance between two routes).

The purpose of conducting experiments using the scientific method is to link the cause (independent variable) to the effect (dependent variable). Scientists then share their results with other scientists, for them to review, to criticize, and ultimately to prove or disprove. Criticism is indispensable for the growth of knowledge, so it is wise to take it with grace. At the end of the process, what was once believed by one individual becomes knowledge shared by a group of people.

The scientific method is used both by scientists and laypeople. The most fundamental aspect of the scientific method is to measure and record. Using our most recent example, a scientist would measure and record the blood pressure levels of two groups of patients taking either green or blue pills. Or a person would measure and record the distance of two routes.

Measuring blood pressure level or distance only one time is not *representative*, meaning it is not the *truth*. The result needs to be observed on multiple occasions. Thus, multiple blood pressure levels will need to be taken from patients randomized to either the set taking the green pill or those taking the blue pill. Similarly, multiple distances will need to be measured between home and work. The multiple values then will need to be averaged to get a mean. It is all about comparing and relating values in cross-sectional (descriptive) or longitudinal (experimental) designs.

The Stats of the Matter

Statisticians deal with studying cause and effect by comparing and relating variables. Statistics is a branch of math, math is a branch of language, and language is a domain of the communicative force.

Referring to the most recent example, statistics is the science that analyzes data—for example, the differences in blood pressure levels between groups or distances between locations. Because single measures from the multiple collections are all over the place, averages or means need to be calculated. The less the variability between each measure, the stronger the relationship. To determine differences between groups (green pill vs blue pill or route 1 vs. route 2), statisticians calculate probabilities. In statistics, the values 0 percent and 100 percent do not exist. It is not even 100 percent certain that one day the sun will come out in the morning.

Statisticians use a mathematical calculation termed P (for probability) *value* to determine if there are significant differences between groups. The aim is to reject falsity. The P value is a number between 0 and 1. (Between, as used here, means that 0 and 1 are not being included.) The P value determines the probability of being wrong. Thus, the lower the P value, the truer the result.

Usually, a P value of ≤ 0.05 (or 5 percent) is considered a significant finding. The 5 percent or less means that the findings have a 1 in 20 chance of being false. (Note: this is a simple example of statistics I am using, but the analyses are much more complex than being explained here.)

Statistics is the most exact science to determine the truth. But as rigorous and systematic as statistics are, it is still peppered with errors. Table 6 shows a few errors encountered in statistics.

Table 6. Sources of errors in statistics	
Population	The population sampled is not representative of the general population (e.g., a study only on patients with hypertension is not representative of the general population).
Sample	The sample recruited at random is skewed (e.g., the green pill group had more patients with severe hypertension).
Season	Seasonal variations exist (e.g., higher blood pressure is more common during holidays).

Instrument	The blood pressure cuff used with the green pill group is off by five millimeters of mercury.
Investigator	Investigator bias exists if the investigator has a personal preference for the blue pill.
Analysis	The analysis methods used may not have been appropriate for this specific study.
Collection	Data collectors may use different methods to measure blood pressure (e.g., some patients were sitting, and others were standing).
Data	Data entry is a cumbersome task and prone to entry mistakes.

The communicative force is the most important creation of the socio-environmental force with the most important feedback being upon the individual. Of all the communicative forces, knowledge is the best tool for personal growth and development. But even with knowledge, every person's decision is still made with some degree of uncertainty.[30]

A person's knowledge expands—to some degree—through repetitive and cumulative processes, and to a large degree, by error elimination. Yet even with this margin of error, humans still land spaceships on planets and build skyscrapers with high precision.

Bibliography

[1] Guyton, A. C., and Hall, J. E. *Textbook of Medical Physiology.* 9th ed. Philadelphia, PA: W. B. Saunders Company, 1996.

[2] Nelson, W. E., and Kliegman, R. M. *Nelson Textbook of Pediatrics.* Philadelphia, PA: Saunders Elsevier Inc., 2004.

[3] Papalia, D. E., Olds, S. W. *A Child's World: Infancy through Adolescence.* 4th ed. New York, NY: McGraw-Hill Inc., 1987.

[4] Pinker, S. *The Language Instinct: How the Mind Creates Language.* New York, NY: HarperCollins Publishers Inc., 1994.

[5] Deacon, T. W. *The Symbolic Species: The Co-Evolution of Language and the Brain.* New York, NY: W. W. Norton & Company, 1997.

[6] Marchant, J. "A journey to the oldest cave paintings in the world" (2016). https://www.smithsonianmag.com/history/journey-oldest-cave-paintings-world-180957685/. Accessed April 5, 2019.

[7] Jean, G. *Writing: The Story of Alphabets and Scripts.* New York, NY: Harry N. Abrams Inc., 1992.

[8] Berwick, R. C., Friederici, A. D., Chomsky, N., and Bolhuis, J. J. "Evolution, brain, and the nature of language." *Trends in Cognitive Sciences* February 2013; 17 (2): 89–98.

[9] Akmajian, A., Demers, R. A., Farmer, A. K., and Harnish, R. M. *Linguistics: An Introduction to Language and Communication.* Cambridge, MA: The MIT Press, 2001.

[10] Onnis, L. "Caregiver communication to the child as moderator and mediator of genes for language." *Behavioural Brain Research* May 15, 2017; 325 (Pt. B): 197–202.

[11] Noble, K. G., McCandliss, B. D., and Farah, M. J. "Socioeconomic gradients predict individual differences in neurocognitive abilities." *Developmental Science* July 2007; 10 (4): 464–480.

[12] Ene, D., Der, G., Fletcher-Watson, S., et al. "Associations of Socioeconomic Deprivation and Preterm Birth With Speech, Language, and Communication Concerns Among Children Aged 27 to 30 Months." *JAMA Network Open* September 4, 2019; 2 (9): e1911027.

[13] Treviño, R. P., Marshall, R. M., Hale, D. E., Rodriguez, R., Baker, G., and Gomez, J. E. "Diabetes risk factors in low-income Mexican-American children." *Diabetes Care* February 1999; 22 (2): 202–207.

[14] Tremblay, P., and Dick, A. S. "Broca and Wernicke are dead, or moving past the classic model of language neurobiology." *Brain and Language* November 2016; 162: 60–71.

15 Ardila, A., Bernal, B., and Rosselli, M. "How Localized are Language Brain Areas? A Review of Brodmann Areas Involvement in Oral Language." *Archives of Clinical Neuropsychology: The Official Journal of the National Academy of Neuropsychologists* February 2016; 31 (1): 112–122.

16 Chang, E. F., Raygor, K. P., and Berger, M. S. "Contemporary model of language organization: an overview for neurosurgeons." *Journal of Neurosurgery* February 2015;122 (2): 250–261.

17 Wilson, S. M., Bautista, A., and McCarron, A. "Convergence of spoken and written language processing in the superior temporal sulcus." *NeuroImage* May 1, 2018; 171: 62–74.

18 Khoshkhoo S, Leonard MK, Mesgarani N, Chang EF. Neural correlates of sine-wave speech intelligibility in human frontal and temporal cortex. *Brain and language.* Dec 2018;187: 83–91.

19 Bouton S, Chambon V, Tyrand, R., et al. Focal versus distributed temporal cortex activity for speech sound category assignment. *Proceedings of the National Academy of Sciences of the United States of America.* Feb 6 2018;115(6): e1299–e1308.

20 Hannagan, T., Amedi, A., Cohen, L., Dehaene-Lambertz, G., and Dehaene, S. "Origins of the specialization for letters and numbers in ventral occipitotemporal cortex." *Trends in Cognitive Sciences* July 2015; 19 (7): 374–382.

21 Purcell, J. J., Jiang, X., Eden, G. F. "Shared orthographic neuronal representations for spelling and reading." *NeuroImage* February 15, 2017; 147: 554–567.

22 Planton, S., Longcamp, M., Peran, P., Demonet, J. F., and Jucla, M. "How specialized are writing-specific brain regions? An fMRI study of writing, drawing and oral spelling." *Cortex; a Journal Devoted to the Study of the Nervous System and Behavior* March 2017; 88: 66–80.

23 Soltanlou, M., Sitnikova, M. A., Nuerk, H. C., and Dresler, T. "Applications of Functional Near-Infrared Spectroscopy (fNIRS) in Studying Cognitive Development: The Case of Mathematics and Language." *Frontiers in Psychology* 2018; 9: 277.

24 Crosson, B. "Thalamic mechanisms in language: a reconsideration based on recent findings and concepts." *Brain and Language* July 2013; 126 (1): 73–88.

25 Llano, D. A. *Neurobiology of Language.* Waltham, MA: Academic Press, 2015.

26 Oh, A., Duerden, E. G., and Pang, E. W. "The role of the insula in speech and language processing." *Brain and Language* August 2014; 135: 96–103.

27 Smith, T., and Osborne, J. H. *Successful Advertising: Its Secret Explained.* London, Eng: Smith's Printing, Publishing and Advertising Agency, 1897.

28 Schmidt, S. "Advertising repetition: A meta-analysis on effective frequency in advertising." *Journal of Advertising* 2015; 44 (4): 415–428.

29 Ford, K. W. *The Quantum World: Quantum Physics for Everyone.* Cambridge, MA: Harvard University Press, 2004.

30 Popper, K. R. *Objective Knowledge: An Evolutionary Approach.* Oxford, England: Oxford University Press, 1979.

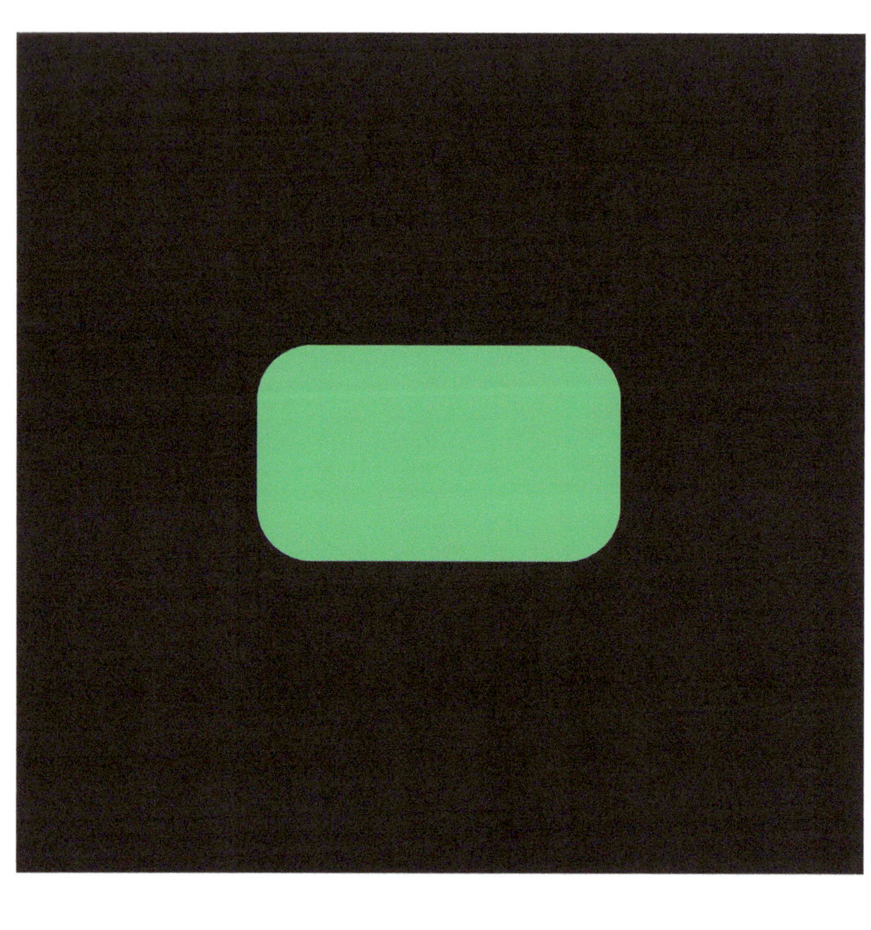

CHAPTER 4

Socio-Environmental Force
The Attraction

The purpose of the socio-environmental force is attraction. Attraction is defined as a natural affinity to objects and living things. There is an unlimited amount of affinity among all objects in the socio-environment. The socio-environmental force tends to cluster objects together into similar groups such as sports teams, race, culture, careers, animal species, religion, politics, professional associations, and the solar system just to name a few. Association comes from the word *associate*, which means "to connect or come together."

In this book, I have divided objects in the socio-environment into two categories: human (socio) and nonhuman (environment). Environment comprises everything from a pebble on the ground to the last galaxy at the edge of the universe.

The socio-environmental force emanates from all objects in the universe. Objects are anything that can be indicated or referred to.[1] They can be social—family, friends, teachers. They can be physical—radios, spoons, cars. Or the objects can be abstract—morals, racism, compassion. Even a person's specific action can be an object. For example, if a person places himself in the position of another or imagines acting in a certain manner, these can become the object for the person.

The socio-environmental force is more closely related to the communicative force than it is to the affective and cognitive forces. Like the communicative force, the socio-environmental force is carried by light, sound, smell, taste, and touch; and its messages are attitudes, beliefs, knowledge, and behaviors. The difference between these forces is that the socio-environmental force creates the messages, which the communicative force then takes and utilizes to get, keep, and increase the four necessities.

As for the ideas being conveyed in the messages, objects like plants and animals emit only attitudes and behaviors that humans like or dislike. A plant that grew green and flowered will produce a positive attitude, and similarly, a dog that learns to sit when told will produce a positive attitude toward the individual. Something traveled between the plant and the individual and the dog and the individual that produced a like or dislike. This something is a force that could be either photons, sound waves, or air fragrances that struck the individual's sense organs. Humans, on the other hand, emit all four: attitudes, beliefs, knowledge, and behaviors.

Matter *Matters*

Humans' affinity for social relations is indispensable to successful living, and as explained in chapter 1, research shows that people who lack relationships die prematurely. People want to be attracted to one another and interact with other beings and nature.

We are social beings, and we are attracted to others. Environmental objects, like social ones, also attract. Stand at the foot of a mountain and look up; walk along the beach and listen to the ocean waves; hike through a forest and smell the fragrance. Without a word or gesture being said or displayed, there is a force being transmitted from these objects that attract us.

Why do people visit a zoo or send *Voyager 1* toward the stars? These objects (the animals, the stars) attract people. It is an affinity empowered by the socio-environmental force. It is animals, people, and things—not mere empty space—that attract us. It is matter that matters to people.

The Force That Binds

What binds an individual to people and things is the socio-environmental force. The socio-environmental force makes objects gravitate toward one another. True, there are some subtleties in the socio-environmental force that might give off the appearance of it being a repulsive force. So yes, a person may have a family member or friend whom he or she doesn't even want to see in person or a photo. And yes, there are some objects that do not attract an individual, like a fire ant or a tree on top of a car. These objects produce stimuli that are aversive. Clustering has its extremes too—for example, Protestants versus Catholics, Muslims versus Jews, and Sunni versus Shiites. But for almost all intents and purposes, the socio-environmental force is an attractive force. Just look at the proliferation of web-based social network applications: Facebook, Myspace, X (formerly known as Twitter), Threads, LinkedIn, eHarmony, and many others. This validates the cohesiveness of the socio-environmental force.

Everyone and Everything Is Related

Objects—people and things—in the socio-environment are relative. By this, I mean what affects one affects the other. Objects are considered in comparison to or in relationship with one another. Thus, the socio-environmental force is a web of relationships and interactions that people weave around themselves. Without this web, life would be meaningless. It would be like an individual floating in space alone, in darkness.

In contrast, the socio-environmental force intertwines objects with the individual. To get the four necessities, the individual moves along the web by comparing and relating one person to another and one thing to another. The individual characterizes each person or thing and then places them into categories.

In characterizing and categorizing, people compare one person to another or compare one thing to another. Many times, people do this kind of operation unknowingly. So for example, over time in her life, a woman may date several men. She will characterize them after meeting them. In her mind, some will be nice and some not so nice, some will be witty and some will be airheaded, some will dress fashionably and some will have no style sense, and some will be quiet and some will be loud. After she makes such comparisons, she may come to choose a future spouse or partner for herself (hopefully not one based on looks alone).

Or a supervisor also will interact with several employees, afterward characterizing them as either hard workers or not, social or antisocial, and skillful or untalented. Then the supervisor will make a choice as to which employee to promote.

By characterizing and categorizing to form comparisons, people gravitate toward certain persons and things in the socio-environment. Such assessments guide the individuals on what paths to take to get, keep, and increase the four necessities.

Relationships and interactions are contingent on a benefit. It could be as simple as gaining status ("I got a new friend") or complex, like gaining wealth ("she got me a job"). Relationships and interactions are interdependent. People consider what each other is hoping to get out of the interaction. We depend on each other. The classic rock group Pink Floyd wrote it better:

Hey You

Hey, you!
Out there in the cold
Getting lonely, getting old.
Can you feel me?

Hey, you!
Standing in the aisles
With itchy feet and fading smiles.
Can you feel me?

Hey, you!
Don't help them to bury the light.
Don't give in without a fight.

Hey, you!
Out there on your own
Sitting naked by the phone.

Would you touch me?

Hey, you!
With your ear against the wall
Waiting for someone to call out.
Would you touch me?

Hey, you!
Would you help me to carry the stone?
Open your heart, I'm coming home

But it was only fantasy.
The wall was too high as you can see.
No matter how he tried he could not break free.
And the worms ate into his brain.

Hey, you!
Out there on the road,
Always doing what you're told.
Can you help me?

Hey, you!
Out there beyond the wall,
Breaking bottles in the hall.
Can you help me?

Hey, you!
Don't tell me there's no hope at all.
Together we stand,
Divided we fall.

The View Matters

The socio-environmental force is physically "out there," but what matters most is what is in there (i.e., in the mind of the individual). It is the individual who chooses what view is important, and he or she perceives the socio-environmental force from his or her own point of view. From this frame of reference, the individual chooses what does or doesn't matter for his or her self-preservation and well-being.

The individual's own attitudes, beliefs, knowledge, and behaviors come into the picture to represent what in the socio-environment is or is not important to him or her. At the moment of observation, the object(s) in the socio-environment and the individual's experiences fuse to create a (distorted) reality. What is out there is important, but more important is how a person feels and thinks once an observation is made. The individual is not a passive receiver. The individual who notes and appraises objects presented to him or her and based on these formulates a response or just a feeling.

People try to mindread one another. They try to anticipate or predict what the other person is feeling, thinking, or intending to do. This *mentalizing* is called the theory of mind. The theory of mind is important to judge and analyze each other's intentions and behaviors. It helps to formulate a response to what is mentalized. Let's say you walk into the kitchen and see your spouse nodding her head and pouting. You mindread that something is wrong and ask how things are. In the previous chapters, we explained how often these exercises can be wrong. But we keep doing it.

Insular Cortex

The insula or insular cortex is the brain processing center of the socio-environmental force. *Insula* means "island" in Latin. The name was given because at one time the insula was isolated from the four main cerebral cortex lobes: frontal, temporal, parietal, and occipital. Although the insula sits under the frontal, temporal, and parietal lobes it has been lifted to the big four as a separate fifth lobe (see figure 1). This upgrade has to do with the new and important role the insula plays in discerning stimuli coming from the socio-environmental force. Particularly, it plays the lead role in the *salience network*.[2] Salience network is a cluster of coordinated brain regions that communicate with each other to select which incoming stimuli from the socio-environment are deserving of attention.

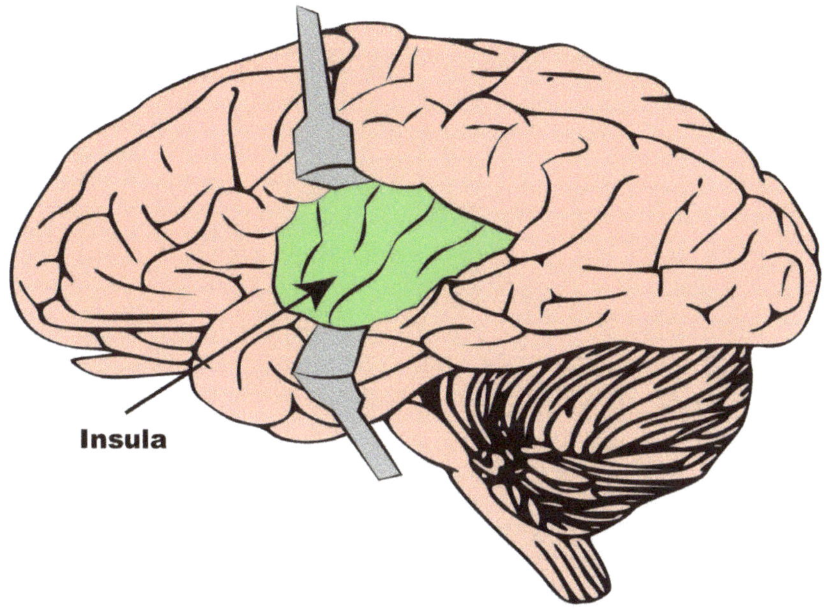

Figure 1. Insular cortex

People are constantly being bombarded by a battery of competing stimuli coming from the socio-environmental force. Just imagine someone driving late to work. The brain is being blitzed by the red light ahead, the blue car too close on the side, the boss calling on the phone, the daughter at home with a fever, the low fuel signal lights up, and on and on. Independent brain structures cannot be shooting off signals simultaneously in different directions to decide and prioritize incoming stimuli. There needs to be one traffic control center. That hub is the insula.

The insula jumps into action when the individual is confronted with complex and uncertain environments, particularly when drastic changes occur in the social environment in which the individual participates. It regulates social interactions and maintains a stable equilibrium of interpersonal relationships. The insula captures both negative (deception, disgust) and positive (compassion, trust) stimuli coming from the social networks in which it participates.[3] These brain processes are often conscious, but they can occur unconsciously.

The main cluster of brain regions that the insula communicates with to execute a response are, as expected, the amygdala, the thalamus, and the cerebral cortex. The stimuli coming from the socio-environmental force can entail social emotion and social cognition operations.[4] When the insula perceives social-emotional stimuli it partners with the amygdala.[5] Whereas the amygdala is considered an impulsive system, the insula is considered a reflective system. When social cognitive stimuli are perceived the insula partners with the thalamus.[6] Whereas the thalamus is responsible for cognitive functions, the insula is responsible for assessing the environment. It is important to note that the insula receives all sensory inputs via the thalamus. The cerebral cortex comes into action once a response is decided.

There is one more anatomical finding to support the insula as the hub for processing stimuli coming from the socio-environmental force. The insula is the only brain structure where von Economo neurons are found. These are large neurons that allow rapid communication across very large brains. An oddity is that these specific neurons are only found in animals known to have large brains and to be social.[7] Of course humans, but these neurons are also found in primates of the hominid lineage such as bonobos, chimpanzees, and gorillas; and in elephants, dolphins, and whales. (Yes, we know about antisocial humans, but as we stated in the introduction, this book is about physiology, not pathophysiology.)

Society

This section will focus on how society has an enormous effect on the individual. (I will discuss the impact of the environment later in this chapter.) Society is people coming together to form a high order of interdependent relationships for the purpose of getting, keeping, and increasing the four necessities of health, wealth, status, and basic drives. Society and individual interact positively and negatively in a reciprocal manner. The individual, though, has a mind of his or her own and has choices when confronted with people and objects.

The individual experiences both social interactions and social relationships.[8] The difference between social interactions and social relationships is a matter of degree, not kind. Interaction is nonintimate, and relationship is intimate. Social interaction occurs when the individual calls a salesperson to ask for the price of merchandise or pays an attendant on duty for gas at a convenience store. Such interactions are important for society to be able to function (people need one another to be able to buy groceries, pay the water bill, deliver a package, reserve a hotel room, board the dog, and on and on).

A relationship occurs when the people-to-people encounters are more frequent, more long-term, and more intimate (i.e., those experienced with a spouse, parent, family member, friend, peer, colleague, and acquaintance). The closer is the relationship the stronger is the attraction. Siblings will have a stronger attraction than will an individual and an acquaintance. Interpersonal relationships are described by their general level of intimacy in table 1.

Table 1. Different types of interpersonal relationships	
Parents	Father, mother, or legal guardian responsible for raising children to their fullest potential
Family	A group of persons related by blood, marriage, or adoption
Intimate Friends	Persons whom one knows, likes, trusts, and confides in
Personal Friends	Persons whom one identifies with because of cultural similarities (professional, ethnic, religious, occupational, trades, social clubs)
Peers	Persons whom one identifies with because of sharing equal "social cells" (work, school, organizations)
Acquaintance	Persons whom one knows

In a relationship, people are constantly searching for persons who can validate and support their core attitudes, beliefs, knowledge, and behaviors. These core constructs are stored in memory; are learned through experiences; are taught by imitating; and serve as tools an individual uses to get, keep, and increase his or her four necessities. Any rejection of an individual's core constructs by people with whom he/she has a close relationship may cause great distress to the individual and could even be a reason for that person to terminate the relationship.

Most relationships between the individual and society are conditional and reciprocal. Both have ideas about what kind of relationship they want and what they plan to obtain from it. At the core, each is looking to get, keep, and increase the four necessities. The individual seeks the potential of satisfying his or her own necessities and understands what he or she needs to do to satisfy the necessities of the other. These are synergistic relationships, and they are the most common of relationships.

Antagonistic relationships occur when one takes advantage of the other without giving anything in return. Altruistic relationships, which are of the highest order, are when a human contributes to the welfare of other people without expecting anything in return. Although the relationship between the individual and society is two-way, or bidirectional, the strong effect society has on the individual cannot be ignored.

A person is highly interdependent on society to satisfy his or her four necessities. Without a safe neighborhood in which to walk, a nearby pool in which to swim, or a local market in which to buy fruits and vegetables, an individual may not have the means to be and stay healthy. Without being taught the value of an education, the value of a good work ethic, and the value of saving, the individual may not have the means to attain wealth. So society provides an individual with the means to tend to the four necessities.

Whether or not the individual tends to the four necessities depends on the kind of socialization he or she receives while growing up. Fulfilling the four necessities provides a person with the maximum amount of joy possible and is a prerequisite for well-being.

Providing More Good Than Bad

A human is born helpless. Other than some basic reflexes needed for survival (suction, grasp, and cry), a baby has no other means to tend to his or her four necessities. Through socialization, however, the child integrates into society, and society then displays by role modeling or by teaching the means of how to tend to the four necessities.

Socialization is the process by which parents, teachers, friends, peers, religious leaders, and many others show or teach the child ideals for how to be successful. Through this process society may show or instruct the child on how to be an engineer or how to be a car thief; it depends on how society raises him or her.

If a child is raised in a community where most go to college, then he or she has a higher likelihood of going to college than a child raised in a community where most don't.[9] If a young woman is raised in a community where most teenagers get pregnant, then she has a higher likelihood of getting pregnant than if she is raised in a community where most do not.

Fortunately, more good than bad has occurred from socialization. The proof is that throughout the millions of years of evolution, humans' physical (many Olympic records keep getting broken) and mental (the new technological and scientific discoveries) capabilities have advanced to outstanding levels.

There may only be four necessities, but the means to fulfill them constitute a million (or more) ways. Humans are born with a large brain capacity to learn what society has available for them. From a child's birth on, he or she experiences social institutions ready to mold and place him or her into a social position. Family, schools, work, church, government, media, and many others are the social institutions; plumber, seamstress, banker, homeless man, burglar, student, and many others are the social positions.

The Impact of Social Institutions and Society

It may be easy to think that the intention of social institutions is to always accommodate the individual into finding or attracting positive social positions. Yet this is not always the case. A broken family may produce a school dropout, a school counselor may discourage a student from attending college, or a workplace may not promote a perfectly qualified employee. So social institutions can direct the individual to take a favorable or unfavorable social position.

Social institutions are what socializes the individual. The individual's personality—which is comprised of attitudes, beliefs, knowledge, and behaviors—are not inherited traits but instead are traits developed by the process of socialization. The individual may have some biological predispositions; but how others act toward him or her, what they teach him or her, and the opportunities society presents to him or her have a greater impact than biological predispositions on what social position he or she assumes.

Socialization means that the individual adopts the qualities and acceptable behaviors that society imposes on him or her. Society influences the individual's feelings, thinking, and behavior and controls and guides the individual's responses. (These are called norms.)

Through rewards and punishments, society teaches the individual how and when to behave. A person may have a certain inclination of how to behave when incited by an event or thing, but the behavior manifested is usually what is deemed "socially acceptable." Societal influences color people's perceptions (i.e.,). Even how the individual sees is filtered by whatever experiences society has shown or taught him or her. So how the individual views him or herself and views others is subtly socially engineered.

The Familial Influence

Family is the social institution responsible for a person's primary socialization. All other social institutions (school, work, government, commerce, churches, et al.) are secondary. While parenting is instinctual to all animals, humans require something beyond what animals need: special skills, which go hand-in-hand with a level of maturity.[10]

Parenting is the cornerstone for children to be raised with the potential to reach their fullest capabilities. If parenting is adequate from the beginning, children are more likely to grow up with the appropriate capabilities to get, keep, and increase the four necessities. Parenting gives the child his or her first foundation in terms of societal values, norms, and rules. Raising a child is a fine balance between love (positive reinforcement) and discipline (negative reinforcement). This love and discipline must be delivered in a most consistent manner.[11] Too much love may spoil the child; too much discipline may traumatize the child. Too lenient discipline can lose its effect, and too forceful or brutal discipline can produce antisocial behaviors in a child. It is a fine balance.

Discipline is something you do for a child; punishment is something you do to a child. Discipline must be accompanied by an explanation and corrective advice. Good parenting also teaches self-control so a child can keep a check on his or her desires and passions.

A parent's rejection of his or her child has been shown to correlate strongly with antisocial behavior in that child.[12, 13] Antisocial behavior is when an individual repetitively and intentionally causes harm to another member of society. Studies have shown that children raised with disrupted mother-infant bonding or in fatherless households have been associated more frequently with affectionless or psychopathic or criminal behaviors.[14] Even in a two-parent household, children can still develop antisocial behaviors if the child is raised by parents who provide harsh and inconsistent discipline, little or no positive reinforcers, or poor or no supervision.[15]

Antisocial behavior is most likely a developmental trait, and less likely a genetic trait. Unfortunately, a child has no say as to what environment he or she is born into or to which parents he or she is born.

Peer Impact

Another member of society who has a great influence on a person is his or her peers.[16] When a person experiences rejection or bullying by his or her peers, it can be cause for the development of antisocial tendencies.

In the United States, a recent phenomenon is a youth walking into a school with firearms and opening fire on students and teachers. One precipitating factor here is the increased bullying among peers (a facilitating factor is the nation's permissive gun culture). Bullying is when a more powerful member of society repetitively causes physical or verbal harm to a less powerful member. Bullying among school-aged youth is now being recognized as a problem affecting the social function of youth. Those who are constantly bullied will develop poorer psychosocial adjustment and have greater difficulty making friends. And on occasion, those being bullied repetitively may retaliate with an extremely aggressive act, such as a mass shooting.[17]

Social Circumstances

Adverse social circumstances—such as living in poor neighborhoods, recondite government policies, or attending substandard schools—can impact a person's behaviors and biology.[18, 19] Children living in socially-deprived neighborhoods have been shown to have a higher risk for antisocial behaviors.[18] This risk is heightened particularly among middle-school children, which is an age when children go through critical biological and psychological development.[20] People living in poor neighborhoods also have a three-fold increase in type 2 diabetes rates compared to those living in affluent neighborhoods.[21]

Government and schools can have a negative effect on the individual. The US Department of Agriculture (USDA) gives schools cash and commodities to help cover the cost of the National School Lunch Program (NSLP) and School Breakfast Program (SBP) meals.[22] In 2009, the USDA reimbursement to the schools for a free priced NSLP meal was $2.57 while the cost to produce it was $2.92. Not much has changed since then and operating at a deficit means that many schools cannot provide quality nutrients in their school lunches for the students. Moreover, on several occasions, the commodities the USDA gives to the schools are those high in fat, sugar, and salt.

Not only can the nutrients afforded be of low quality but the children are also rushed to have their lunch period done within twenty minutes. Children eating rushed meals are more likely to consume lower quality food and higher plate waste.[23, 24] In these ways, government and schools can negatively affect children's health, for children are eating less-than-recommended fruits and vegetables in many elementary schools.[25, 26] Plus, once the children get to middle school, taking a physical education class is no longer a requirement and recess has been discontinued in most US schools.[27] All these constitute a recipe for unhealthy behaviors.

The cause of chronic disease in special populations thus may not be a biological predisposition—as is usually thought to be—but more an imbalance of the social milieu in which the populations are embedded. As many studies show, the attraction that the individual has toward other members of society does not always produce favorable results.

Reciprocal Interactions

When the individual interacts with the socio-environment, the interaction is not unidirectional but bidirectional.[9] At the point of interaction, the individual and socio-environment both have an effect on each other. Both become one and inseparable as they spin around each other to modify and shape each other. So for example, children can have a great influence on parents and schools, and the parents and schools can have a great influence on children.

Let's look at it this way: A newborn child changes his or her parents' life in ways too numerous to count. Instead of going out to the movies, parents may watch movies at home; instead of staying up late, parents may go to bed early to catch up on lost or interrupted sleep; and instead of eating out, parents may start cooking at home to attend their child's nutritional needs and not disrupt other diners by bringing a newborn with them to a restaurant.

If school-aged children are not eating the cafeteria food, then the schools will change the menu; if the children are behind in math, then schools will change the way they are teaching the children math; and if the children experience many disciplinary problems, then schools will provide more counseling. The influence therefore of parents and schools on children (and vice versa!) is obvious.

From Four Legs to Two

The individual and socio-environmental attraction is reciprocal in that each can affect and change the other. For the most part, this reciprocal interaction has been positive. It is the interaction that has propelled humans upward (from four legs to two legs) and also forward (from stones to silicon).

Culture

Now that I've explained how society affects the individual within his or her present generation,[9] let's discuss how society affects the individual from one generation to the next. Culture is a pattern of attitudes, beliefs, knowledge, and behaviors that society transmits to the individual across and down generational lines. The cultural patterns that are accepted by society are the customs the individual usually adopts to get, keep, and increase the four necessities. These are the tools the individual uses to get what he or she desires from society and are also what society needs to get from the individual for him or her to be a productive member of the group. The adoption and transmission of these customary cultural practices are important for the continuation of society in an orderly fashion.

Culture influences human actions because of its attitudes, beliefs, knowledge, and behavioral foundations, as usually, a person will behave according to what he or she thinks and feels. So if the individual with a family history of diabetes believes that exercising is healthy and knows that walking 150 minutes a week is enough to prevent diabetes, then it is likely that this person will establish a weekly walking routine. It is also possible that this way of thinking will be passed on to future generations along family lines, either by direct instruction or by role modeling. It is also possible that through the transmittal of this way of thinking, the chances of future generations of family members getting diabetes can be minimized or stopped altogether.[28]

An Orderly Set

Culture is the soup that keeps all the ingredients together. Culture consists of a system of attitudes, beliefs, knowledge, and behaviors that come together to compose values, norms, and rules. Values and norms are more belief-based, and rules are more knowledge-based. Values and norms are informal standards of conduct, and rules are formal standards of conduct imposed by society on the individual.

Values are a way of thinking or a set of ideas that the individual is taught as being right or wrong or as being important or not important. So the individual may value one political system over another, one religion over another, one economic system over another, or some family customs over others. If a neighborhood values historical preservation, for example, then it is more likely for the residents to restore their homes to their original design. If parents value frugality, then they expect their children to turn off the lights and water faucets when not in use. Values tend to be passed along generational lines.

Norms are a set of understandings that lay the framework for how the individual should behave in public. Norms are a way of acting imposed on the individual by wider societal demands. The purpose of having norms is to permit people to live together without them encroaching on each other's possessions and rights. By delineating what is permissible and what is forbidden, norms keep society functioning in an orderly fashion. Some common societal norms are not to cut when waiting in line, give up one's chair to an elderly person, hold the elevator or door when another is approaching, and for children be respectful to adults. Norms are informal standards and regulated by loose sanctions.

Rules are more formal and comprise laws, policies, and regulations. Rules grow out of extensive deliberations. They are detailed in written documents and regulated by firm sanctions. Rules are researched and developed by a group of people who specialize in the subject of interest. These persons bring in their sets of knowledge and expertise and, after deliberation, decide what laws, policies, and regulations should be implemented. Once a decision is made as to the rules, the rules are written into codes or manuals. If rules are broken, the individual may lose his or her job, be thrown out of a particular social club, or may even end up in jail.

A System of Rewards and Punishments

Society rewards the individual who conforms and punishes those who violate, set values, norms, and rules. If the individual's thinking (beliefs and knowledge) and behaviors do not adhere to or conform to set values, norms, and rules, then society will reprimand him or her.

Values, norms, and rules are necessary to keep society functioning in an orderly fashion and to keep the individual improving his or her standard of living. Society regulating values, norms, and rules has driven humans to extraordinary levels of self-improvement. Over the millions of years of evolution, humans have become faster and smarter, and they generally live longer lives. In a sense, what society is to the individual, a parent is to a child. Overall, society has done an extraordinary job in raising healthier, wealthier, sociable, and sensible individuals. But it is not all perfect.

Since it is individual thought and behavior that breaks society's values, norms, and rules, the individual should be judged by what he or she thinks and does, and not by how he or she looks, which is often the case. Without having any insight as to the individual's thoughts and behaviors, society may reject that individual purely on outer appearances: "He is fat," "She is ugly," "His eyes are slanted," "Her nose is flat," or "He is too short." Because the individual does not talk like them, look like them, walk like them, or dress like them, then they (society) may reject him or her.

While it is human nature to detest what is different, some manifest it externally whereas others do not, some control it and some do not, and some correct the sectarian pattern of acting and some never stop themselves from acting in this hurtful fashion. Overcoming bigotry takes education, self-reflection, and practicing tolerance.

Memes

Memes are units of information that are transmitted from one mind to another.[29] These are attitudes, beliefs, knowledge, and behaviors that are replicated by means of imitation. Proponents of memes use genes as an analogy—that memes, like genes, are instructions for human development; memes are replicators like genes; memes, like genes, are transmitted from one generation to the next; memes, like genes, are long-lived; memes and genes interact by coevolution; and that memes, like genes, go through the process of natural selection. Accordingly, memes replicate, vary, and the versions that can adapt to socio-environmental pressures are the ones that will be preserved long-term.

There are some gaps in using memes as analogs to gene transmission. Meme theory is not widely accepted in the scientific community.[30] Social scientist view "memetics" as lacking scientific rigor. According to proponents of memes, a brain center is yet to be found.[31] Memes do not have chromosome loci or alleles. Whereas genes are transmitted vertically from one generation to the next, memes are transmitted vertically and horizontally—from a parent to a child and from a worker to a coworker. Lastly, why come up with a new term when one already exists? The term is *culture*. Culture "bytes" do have specific storage sites in the brain. These are called memory engrams. In chapter 2, "Cognitive Force," we described the memory engram, whose function and location have been observed.[32]

A memory engram is an ensemble of neurons that store related attitudes, beliefs, knowledge, and behaviors in a cluster of related synapses. Memory engrams are traces of long-term memory consolidated in the brain. This collection of specialized neurons undergoes persistent chemical and physical changes to become an engram. The attitudes, beliefs, knowledge, and behaviors in memory engrams can be taught by imitation; and when the receiver uptakes these, they will vary some to adapt to the receiver's point of view. Memory engrams are experiences learned from the socio-environment and are useful to get, keep, and increase the four necessities. (Caution: necessities can be negative [e.g., wealth obtained by criminal activity]).

A Culture of Poverty

A culture of poverty is characterized by inept patterns of thinking and behaving that are transmitted like genes along family lines.[33] It is a way of life that is stable and persistent and passed from one generation to the next along family lines.

A culture of poverty, along it being self-inflicted, can also be transmitted by the socio-environmental force. Parents did not teach him good work ethics, or the employer will not hire her because she is not dressed fashionably. The individual born into a culture of poverty inherits faulty patterns of thinking and behaving that may cripple him or her from getting, keeping, and increasing his or her four necessities.

Please note that the culture of poverty has nothing to do with the working or farming class. Nor does it have anything to do with those who had an economic mishap and ended up poor. The people in these particular groups have a different system of thinking and behaving than those in the culture of poverty. The culture of poverty only applies to individuals that, because of faulty patterns of thinking and behaving, remain in the lower socioeconomic status of their own society for at least two generations of family lines.

The culture of poverty implants in the individual some universal characteristics that transcend national and racial/ethnic borders. These individuals spend more energy on their immediate problems and less on planning for the future. They spend most of their time and resources attaining essential needs like food, shelter, clothes, medical care, childcare, or family support and less on planning for the future through getting a higher education, building wealth, or living healthy now to prevent disease later.

To relieve stress, humans need immediate gratification. Because of this immediate need, people who inherit the culture of poverty are less likely to sacrifice present pleasures for future rewards. To relieve their stress, wealthy people may take a trip to a foreign country or the beach; but for people living in poverty, their only stress relief may be to overeat and sleep. The latter behaviors in excess predispose such impoverished people to higher rates of chronic disease.[34]

Because of this transmitted cultural disability, people in the culture of poverty will most likely suffer from disproportionate rates of medical, financial, social, and personal problems. For example, diabetes is a medical problem suffered mostly by people living in poverty.[21] Although diabetes is transmitted along family lines, scientists assume that a defective gene plays a major role in the cause. My position on this is that genes do not command what a society becomes; social interactions and culture do.

In the Western world, many scientists are overly influenced by outdated mechanic physics, wherein all effects are attempted to be reduced to one sole cause. Well, human behavior is more like quantum physics, where multiple causes interact to produce one effect. Yet because of Western civilization's reductionist scientific methods, our society spends enormous amounts of time and resources searching for defective genes or miracle drugs, and less on modifying the socio-environment that influences health (home, neighborhoods, schools, commerce, government).

More than Just the Individual

The culture of poverty is not just an individual problem; it is also a societal problem. The culture of poverty is a product of two forces: individual choice and societal imposition. The individual proposes, and society imposes.

People exposed to the culture of poverty have difficulty adjusting to society's demands, and in return, society tends to reject these people. The culture of poverty has its own social characteristics and its own distinctive consequences that affect the individual and the wider society in which he or she is embedded. These circumstances lead to an endless loop of poverty and illiteracy that can last for generations. Low education levels stem from the fact that education in the Western hemisphere is very expensive. This causes people from lower income brackets to resist college-level education.

Low income and low education levels stifle the individual from attaining the four necessities; and without wealth, health, status, and basic drive fulfillment, the individual cannot pull him or herself out of the culture of poverty. Individuals who "inherit" the culture of poverty usually keep themselves—and are also kept by society—on the lower rungs of the economic ladder. Society suffers economic losses, too, when this happens. Society ends up paying more for housing, food, and medical care through higher taxes. Thus, the culture of poverty is a vicious cycle produced by both the individual and society.

When some members of society are asked why some people fall into the culture of poverty, their response may be "Because they are lazy," "Because they are ignorant," "Because they cannot hold a job," or "Because they just want to live off welfare." In other words, some members of society do not see this culture as a product of wider societal influences. Yet indeed this can be the cause.

Let me use what I term the unemployment cascade as an example. When the unemployment rate goes down, businesses will pay more for salaries because of decreased labor force → high salaries then cause inflation → because of high inflation, the Federal Reserve increases interest rates → when interest rates go up, lending goes down → because of high cost to borrow, businesses invest less → lower investment leads to less production → this leads to layoffs. Being laid off is a gate to the culture of poverty.

Another example is the low opportunities given to people living in a culture of poverty. Because these people are more likely to lack wealth, status, and health and may well be of a different ethnicity than those doing the hiring, they are less likely to fare well at job interviews. We are all interdependent on one another.

Environment

The environment has a high degree of attraction, or appeals to, the individual. Houses, flowers, sunsets, animals, gems, mountains, rainbows, and oceans are just a few of a billion environmental objects that enthrall humans. The environment, like society, has a great influence on how humans evolve; and humans also have a great influence on how the environment evolves. Because they need each other, they attract. What connects them both is the socio-environmental force.

Our environment is divided into two large categories: natural environment and built environment. The *natural environment* is objects not created by humans, such as rain, bison, national parks, and galaxies. The *built environment* is objects created by humans, such as highways, buildings, parks, and neighborhoods.

Most humans consider themselves as being part of, or connected to, the natural environment. This feeling of connectedness to the natural environment is a big reason why most people act to conserve and care for nature. When people are asked in surveys to describe their feelings toward the natural environment, they provide words like *tranquil, stunning, pristine, beautiful,* and *peaceful.*[35] When asked to describe the built environment, they offer words like *pollution, waste, crowding, factories,* and *noisy.* The individual and the environment need each other.

Human behavior has created the built environment, and the built environment has influenced human behavior. The arrow going from human to built environment is quite obvious, but how the built environment influences human behavior is still unclear.

According to the Centers for Disease Control and Prevention, a lack of sidewalks and walking and bicycle trails in poorly designed neighborhoods contribute to sedentary behaviors.[36] Sedentary behaviors are a major cause of obesity, cardiovascular disease, diabetes, and other chronic diseases. Several systematic reviews of longitudinal studies conducted around the world found strong causal relationships between the built environment and diseases such as obesity, diabetes, and cardiovascular disease.[37–39] Factors in the built environment that contribute to disease are lack of neighborhood walkability, uncontrolled expansion of urban areas (urban sprawl), excess traffic, and high residential density. Similar to the association between poorly built environments and disease are poor-quality food environments (i.e., food desserts) and disease.[40, 41]

Yes, the individual and environment need each other, but the individual needs the environment more than the environment needs the individual. Through the following sections, I will demonstrate how the environment attracts the individual. Objects in the environment that attract the individual are exhaustive, but to simplify my message, I will use four: water, fire, plants, and animals.

Water

People have a tremendous affinity for water. Go half a day without water, and you'll experience the insatiable thirst! In turn, water needs people in terms of no pollution. Without water, humans could not live; and without water, the earth could not support life. If the atmosphere did not carry water, life would not have crawled out of the sea.

Rain is water transmuting through a circular cycle.[42] The cycle includes water either in the form of ice, liquid, or vapor. (Temperature is one of the factors that determine whether a substance is ice, liquid, or vapor.) A water molecule never dies; it just goes around and around in a perpetual cycle. Water in the form of liquid and the form of ice is visible and measurable. Water in the form of vapor is the invisible gaseous form of water that is always present in the air.

Although invisible and unmeasurable, water vapor exerts the most powerful effect on humans. Water vapor provides the moisture needed for rainbows, clouds, dew, drizzle, fog, frost, rain, snow, thunderstorms, tornadoes, and hurricanes. Hurricanes, as feared and catastrophic as they may be, sometimes are the only means to relieve the dreaded effects of summer droughts seen in the southwestern United States. Without much-needed rain, farmers grow limited produce for human consumption and people restrict water for personal consumption. Thus, rain, in its different presentations, is indispensable for plants and animals to survive.

The amount of water in the human body ranges from 50 percent to 75 percent and the earth's surface has nearly the same amount of water (~70 percent). More than 97 percent of the earth's water is in the ocean as salt water. If 1,000 milliliters were to be equated to all the world's water, 965 milliliters would be in the ocean as salt water and 35 milliliters would be inland as fresh water. Of the 35 milliliters inland, 17 milliliters would be ice and snow, 16 milliliters would be underground (aquifers), 1 milliliter would be rivers and lakes, and 1 milliliter would be in soil and air. Evaporation of just a small portion of the ocean and the atmospheric movement of that water vapor inland are what started the biological evolution of life.

While the cycle of water evaporating and falling as rain balances out over large areas and long periods of time, precipitation at particular places can be high enough to cause floods and low enough to cause droughts. Floods kill more people each year than hurricanes, tornadoes, or lightning. Droughts are and have always been a big part of world history. The longest rainless period in the US was 767 days (Bagdad, California), and in the world, it was fourteen consecutive years (1903 to 1918, Arica, Chile).

In sum, humans have an immense affinity for water, but too much or too little water can be a devastating killer. The coexistence of water and humans is a fine balance.

Fire

The sun is an immense ball of fire with a surface temperature of 3.5 million degrees Fahrenheit (2 million degrees centigrade). Humans not only have an affinity for this ball of fire but they also have worshiped it.

Most of us find it enjoyable to hear the weatherman say, "Tomorrow will be a sunny day." Or when going on vacation or spending a weekend at the beach, people universally feel they will experience no better weather than if they get a sunny day.

The sun and earth have coexisted for four and a half billion years. Without the light from the sun, life on earth would not be possible. The light came first, and matter is a consequence of that light. This is a reality recognized by the very earliest civilizations. Egyptians, Aztecs, and Incas worshipped the sun because they understood that without it, there would be no rain, no crops, and no life.

The sun radiates an invisible energy that affects a person physically and emotionally. Too much sun can cause skin cancer; too little can cause bone disease. A dark cloudy day can set the stage for a person's gloomy mood, and a bright sunny day can inspire a positive mood. The sun provides the earth with the highest level of energy that affects humans and all living things in more than one way.

All living things on earth are powered by the sun's energy. The sun bathes the earth with a wide variety and different amounts of energy. Most of the sun's energy comes in the form of visible light, ultraviolet rays, X-rays, microwaves, and radio waves. It is the sun's ultraviolet rays that provide humans with vitamin D. Without vitamin D your bones would crack like dry tree limbs.

The sun produces energy by using a chemical process called nuclear fusion. In contrast to this, atomic bombs cause the explosion by another chemical process called nuclear fission. Fusion reaction fuses atoms together to give off energy and fission reaction splits atoms apart to produce energy. Like bombs, nuclear plants operate by fission reaction. A big difference exists between natural and man-made nuclear reactions!

The earth's year-long trip around the sun creates the weather. The sun's electromagnetic energy and infrared energy flow into the atmosphere to warm the air, oceans, and land. The result is the earth shares an extremely frigid polar cold and a hot tropical heat. This sets up a heat engine in the earth's atmosphere that powers the weather.

A heat engine depends on hot-cold contrasts to produce power. If we use the car as an example here, the vehicle's engine power comes from the heat created by burning a mixture of gasoline and air in a cylinder. As the engine runs, its cylinders alternate between being hot and cold producing power. The bigger the contrast between hot and cold, the more power it produces. It is similar to what happens in the earth's atmosphere. The greater the hot-cold contrast, the stronger the energy that is released. The same holds true for storms. The greater the hot-cold contrast, the stronger the storm.

Like all matter in the socio-environment, humans and the sun are interconnected, and what affects one affects the other. The sun affects humans enormously, but humans can also affect the sun's influence on earth. Humans can affect the sun's effect on earth's atmosphere by destroying the delicate balance that exists in the atmosphere. Excessive use of manufacturing and automobiles produces greenhouse gases such as ozone and creates a carbon footprint (i.e., higher levels of CO_2 in the atmosphere). This causes the sun's heat to be trapped in the earth's surface causing temperatures to soar above 100 degrees Fahrenheit. The presence of high heat on the earth's surface then causes a gradual melting of the polar ice caps resulting in a surfeit of water in the oceans. An increase in warm water in the oceans results in devastating hurricanes.

Greenhouse destruction is a result of too much carbon dioxide and other human-made gases. The greenhouse effect is important because it traps the sun's heat in the lower atmosphere to keep the earth warm. Like everything in life, the greenhouse effect needs to operate in a fine balance. A moderate greenhouse effect is indispensable for life on earth, but an elevated greenhouse effect is dangerous. An elevated greenhouse effect traps excessive heat, which in turn causes global warming. Some of the harmful effects of global warming on the socio-environment are rising sea levels, drought, flooding, wildfires, and other natural disasters. The coexistence of fire and humans is a fine balance!

Plants

Plants and humans attract each other. Just think of the joy you feel when you see the flowers blossoming in spring. The lack of attraction between plants and individuals can be fatal. Plants die if not watered by humans, and humans die if not nurtured by plants. Table 2 gives twenty-one many reasons why humans can die if they do not consume plants. Plants are a rich source of the vitamins and minerals we need to live. Vitamins are organic foods the body needs to grow and regenerate. Minerals are inorganic elements that cells need to function properly.

Table 2. List of vitamins and minerals plants provide to humans to sustain life	
Vitamins	Minerals
Vitamin A	Calcium
Vitamin B1	Copper
Vitamin B2	Iodine
Vitamin B5	Iron
Vitamin B6	Magnesium
Vitamin B9	Manganese
Vitamin C	Phosphorus
Vitamin D	Potassium
Vitamin E	Selenium
Vitamin K	Sodium
	Zinc

Animals

Humans originated from animals. The animals that had the greatest influence on mankind are the great ape family. Without this animal, humans would have never gotten off the ground.

The hominid, the first ancestor of humans, had both ape and human features. The first known hominid is the *Sahelanthropus tchadensis*, estimated to have lived nearly 7 million years ago (see picture).[43] The distinguishing feature that led to the evolution of apes to hominids was the transition from quadrupedal to bipedal. It was not, as many might believe, the brain. The *Sahelanthropus* brain was not any much different than that of the ape.

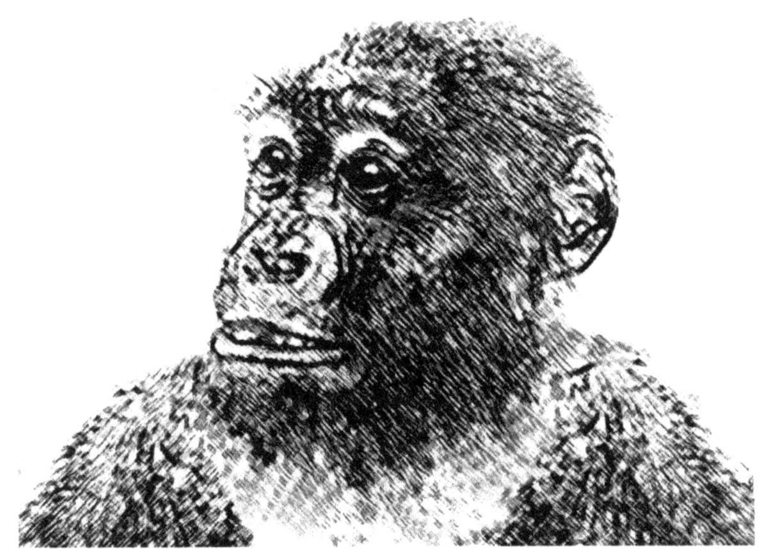

The theory explaining bipedalism has evolved from natural selection to female selection. Bipedalism, it is speculated, was tied to monogamy.[44] As the environment became more seasonal and variable, it became harder to find food. Because raising their babies became more difficult, therefore, females began depending more on males to gather food for themselves and their offspring. Males who had the ability to free their arms and hands could carry more provisions. This led females to begin selecting males who could keep their hands free as they walked, over their knuckle-walking counterparts. It became food-for-mating provisioning.

From seven million to three hundred thousand years ago, hominids stood at the top of the animal kingdom. For this prolonged period, animals and humans were one and the same. It wasn't until three hundred thousand years ago that *Homo sapiens* evolved in Africa, and between sixty thousand and eighty thousand years ago *Homo sapiens* began leaving Africa to populate the rest of the world.[45] *Homo sapiens* would go on to develop a complex brain system and the most sophisticated civilization ever known in the universe.

Individual Determination

The socio-environmental force, because of its attraction, has a big influence on the individual. But of all the forces, the socio-environment is the weakest to influence human behavior. The reason is that the affective, cognitive, and communicative forces are inherent in the individual and the socio-environment is external to the individual. At the end of the day, it is all about the choices the individual makes in life. The individual can either choose to get up at six in the morning to go for a jog or at ten in the morning to have a big breakfast. The choice is up to the individual.

Bibliography

1 Blumer H. *Symbolic interactionism: perspective and method.* Berkeley, CA: University of California Press; 1969.

2 Seeley WW. The Salience Network: A Neural System for Perceiving and Responding to Homeostatic Demands. *J Neurosci.* 2019;39(50):9878-9882.

3 Allman JM, Tetreault NA, Hakeem AY, Park S. The von Economo neurons in apes and humans. *Am J Hum Biol.* 2011;23(1):5-21.

4 González-Acosta CA, Escobar MI, Casanova MF, Pimienta HJ, Buriticá E. Von Economo Neurons in the Human Medial Frontopolar Cortex. *Front Neuroanat.* 2018;12:64.

5 Namkung H, Kim SH, Sawa A. The Insula: An Underestimated Brain Area in Clinical Neuroscience, Psychiatry, and Neurology. *Trends Neurosci.* 2017;40(4):200-207.

6 Zhou K, Zhu L, Hou G, et al. The Contribution of Thalamic Nuclei in Salience Processing. *Front Behav Neurosci.* 2021;15:634618.

7 López-Ojeda W, Hurley RA. Von Economo Neuron Involvement in Social Cognitive and Emotional Impairments in Neuropsychiatric Disorders. *J Neuropsychiatry Clin Neurosci.* 2022;34(4):302-306.

8 Miell D, Dallos R. *Social interaction and personal relationships.* Thousand Oaks, CA: The Open University, Sage Publication; 1996.

9 Kornblum W. Sociology *in a changing world.* 4th ed. Fort Worth, TX: Hardcourt Brace College Publishers; 1997.

10 Papalia DE, Olds SW. *A child's world: infancy through adolescence.* 4th ed. New York, NY: McGraw-Hill, Inc.; 1987.

11 Dobson J. *The new dare to discipline.* Carol Stream, IL: Tyndale House Publishers; 1996.

12 Fuchs A, Mohler E, Reck C, Resch F, Kaess M. The Early Mother-to-Child Bond and Its Unique Prospective Contribution to Child Behavior Evaluated by Mothers and Teachers. *Psychopathology.* 2016;49(4):211-216.

13 Schwartz JA, Wright EM, Valgardson BA. Adverse childhood experiences and deleterious outcomes in adulthood: A consideration of the simultaneous role of genetic and environmental influences in two independent samples from the United States. *Child abuse & neglect.* 2019;88:420-431.

14 Murray J, Farrington DP, Sekol I. Children's antisocial behavior, mental health, drug use, and educational performance after parental

incarceration: a systematic review and meta-analysis. *Psychol Bull.* 2012;138(2):175-210.

15 Waller R, Gardner F, Hyde LW. What are the associations between parenting, callous-unemotional traits, and antisocial behavior in youth? A systematic review of evidence. *Clin Psychol Rev.* 2013;33(4):593-608.

16 Calkins SD, Keane SP. Developmental origins of early antisocial behavior. *Development and psychopathology.* 2009;21(4):1095-1109.

17 Nansel TR, Overpeck M, Pilla RS, Ruan WJ, Simons-Morton B, Scheidt P. Bullying behaviors among US youth: prevalence and association with psychosocial adjustment. *JAMA.* 2001;285(16):2094-2100.

18 Ingoldsby EM, Shaw DS. Neighborhood contextual factors and early-starting antisocial pathways. *Clinical child and family psychology review.* 2002;5(1):21-55.

19 Treviño RP. *Forgotten children: a true story of how politicians endanger children.* San Antonio, TX: Presa Publishing LLC; 2009.

20 Treviño RP. Economic analysis of treating and preventing type 2 diabetes implications for Latino families. In: Perez-Escamilla, R. , Melgar-Quiñonez, H., eds. *At Risk: Latino Children's Health.* Houston, TX: Arte Publico Press; 2011.

21 Burke JP, Williams K, Gaskill SP, Hazuda HP, Haffner SM, Stern MP. Rapid rise in the incidence of type 2 diabetes from 1987 to 1996. *Arch Intern Med.* 1999;159:1450-1456.

22 Treviño RP, Pham T, Mobley C, Hartstein J, El Ghormli L, Songer T. Healthy study school food service revenue and expense report. *Journal of School Health.* 2012;82:417-423.

23 Bergman EA, Buergel NS, Englund TF, Femrite A. The relationship between the length of the lunch period and nutrient consumption in elementary school lunch setting. The Journal of Child Nutrition & Management. 2004(2):http://docs.schoolnutrition.org/newsroom/jcnm/04fall/bergman/bergman02.asp.

24 Cohen JF, Jahn JL, Richardson S, Cluggish SA, Parker E, Rimm EB. Amount of Time to Eat Lunch Is Associated with Children's Selection and Consumption of School Meal Entrée, Fruits, Vegetables, and Milk. J Acad Nutr Diet. 2016;116(1):123-128.

25 Treviño RP, Fogt D, Wyatt TJ, Leal-Vasquez L, Sosa ET, Woods C. Diabetes risk, low fitness, and energy insufficiency levels among children from poor families. Journal of the American Dietetic Association. 2008;108:1846-1853.

26 Balvin Frantzen L, Trevino RP, Echon RM, Garcia-Dominic O, DiMarco N. Association between frequency of ready-to-eat cereal consumption, nutrient intakes, and body mass index in fourth- to sixth-grade low-income minority children. J Acad Nutr Diet. 2013;113(4):511-519.

27 Gordon-Larsen P, McMurray RG, Popkin BM. Determinants of adolescent physical activity and inactivity patterns. Pediatrics. 2000;105(6):E83.

28 Treviño RP, Marshall RM, Hale DE, Rodriguez R, Baker G, Gomez JE. Diabetes risk factors in low-income Mexican-American children. Diabetes Care. 1999;22(2):202-207.

29 Blackmore S. The Meme Machine. Oxford England: Oxford University Press; 1999.

30 Isaacs D. Memes. J Paediatr Child Health. 2020;56(4):497-498.

31 Dawkins, R. *The God Delusion.* New York, NY: Harper Collins, 2006.

32 Josselyn, S. A., and Tonegawa, S. "Memory engrams: Recalling the past and imagining the future." *Science* 2020; 367 (6473).

33 Lewis, O. *Los Hijos de Sanchez.* Mexico City, Mexico: Editorial Grijalbo, S. A. de C.V., 1982.

34 Hu, F., Mason, J., Stampfer, M., et al. « Diet, lifestyle, and the risk of type 2 diabetes mellitus in women." *N Eng J Med.* 2001; 345 (11): 790–797.

35 Vining, J., Merrick, M. S., and Price, E. A. "The distinction between humans and nature: human perceptions of connectedness to nature and elements of the natural and unnatural." *Research in Human Ecology* 2002; 15 (1): 1–11.

36 Carlson, S. A., Paul, P., Watson, K. B., Schmid, T. L., and Fulton, J. E. "How reported usefulness modifies the association between neighborhood supports and walking behavior." *Prev Med.* 2016; 91: 76–81.

37 Chandrabose, M., Rachele, J. N., Gunn, L., et al. « Built environment and cardio-metabolic health: systematic review and meta-analysis of longitudinal studies." *Obes Rev.* 2019; 20 (1): 41–54.

38 den Braver, N. R., Lakerveld, J., Rutters, F., Schoonmade, L. J., Brug, J., and Beulens, J. W. J. "Built environmental characteristics and diabetes: a systematic review and meta-analysis." *BMC Medicine.* 2018; 16 (1): 12.

39 Malambo, P., Kengne, A. P., De Villiers, A., Lambert, E. V., and Puoane, T. "Built Environment, Selected Risk Factors and Major Cardiovascular Disease Outcomes: A Systematic Review." *PloS One* 2016; 11 (11): e0166846.

[40] Ford, P. B., and Dzewaltowski, D. A. "Disparities in obesity prevalence due to variation in the retail food environment: three testable hypotheses." *Nutr Rev.* 2008; 66 (4): 216–228.

[41] Rahman, T., Cushing, R. A., and Jackson, R. J. "Contributions of built environment to childhood obesity." *The Mount Sinai Journal of Medicine, New York* 2011; 78 (1): 49–57.

[42] US Department of the Interior, US Geological Survey. "How much water is there on, in, and above the Earth." https://water.usgs.gov/edu/earthhowmuch.html. Published 2019. Accessed April 12, 2019.

[43] Smithsonian National Museum of Natural History. "Sahelanthropus tchadensis." http://humanorigins.si.edu/evidence/human-fossils/species/sahelanthropus-tchadensis. Published 2019. Accessed April 9, 2019.

[44] Lovejoy, C. O. "The origin of man." *Science* 1981; 211 (4480): 341–350.

[45] Smithsonian National Museum of Natural History. "Humans change the world." http://humanorigins.si.edu/human-characteristics/humans-change-world. Published 2019. Accessed April 9, 2019.

Conclusion

It should be of no surprise that the four forces of human nature and the four fundamental forces of physics have similarities. Humans and the socio-environment are made up of atoms—protons, neutrons, and electrons. Like the four fundamental forces that keep atoms and the universe in kilter, the four forces of human nature do the same for the individual and socio-environment. As stated in the introduction, the affective, cognitive, communicative, and socio-environmental forces have correlations with the strong, weak, electromagnetic (EM), and gravity forces, respectively. There is still so much to know and learn about these two fields. And what we know now might change with new scientific discoveries. But in this book, we stayed focused on what we know of neuroscience—specifically, on the amygdala, thalamus, cerebral cortex, and insula or insular cortex. We have described their features and explained their workings. Following are some similarities between the two sets of forces.

Affective Force ≈ Strong Force

The strong force keeps the nucleus together, operates at short distances, and does not work on electrons. It is obvious by the name that the strong force is stronger than the weak force. Similarly, the affective force keeps the individual together, operates as far as a facial or hand expression can reach, and does not work on the communicative force. The affective force is stronger than the cognitive force. In this book, I made the case for how passion triumphs over reason and how impulsivity triumphs over rational thought.

Every morning, when you wake up until the time when you go to sleep, it is the affective force that keeps you safe and healthy. It is the affective force, consciously or subconsciously, that guides you down the stairs to make sure you are kept all together in one piece. As you are driving home from work, it is the affective force that is on the lookout for the red light or the 18-wheeler speeding up the intersection.

The processing center of the affective force is the amygdala. The amygdala is the first responder, and in times of emergency, it over-rules the thalamus. The amygdala is like oxygen, and the thalamus is like water. Humans can survive for hours without water but will die within minutes without oxygen. Lastly, the affective force does not work on the communicative force. It is the cognitive force that links with the communicative force as a unified higher learning process that involves reason and language.

Cognitive Force ≈ Weak Force

The weak force, like the cognitive force, is complex and needs more explanation. The weak force is responsible for decay and trans-mutation, emits radiation, operates at longer distances, and works on the nucleus and electrons. Similarly, the cognitive force is responsible for transforming the individual, emits radiation, operates at longer distances, and works on the affective and communicative forces.

Decay in physics does not mean food rotting or decomposing. It means that particles go through reactions that transform them into other particles—for example, carbon being transformed into nitro-gen or phosphorus into sulfur. Transmutation, like decay, is the con-version of one element into another.

Another process of the weak force is radioactivity. Radioactivity is the emission of light. Light, rays, radiation, and photons are one and the same. Light—like rays, radiation, and photons—carry energy; and this energy can be loaded with bundles of information and transmitted as waves/particles.

The weak force has a farther reach than the strong force. Whereas the strong force works only with the nucleus, the weak force works with the nucleus and electrons. Photons are the weak force messengers that go back and forth between the nucleus and electrons carrying bundles of information.

The processing center of the cognitive force is the thalamus. The thalamus works with the amygdala and cerebral cortex to perform cognitive functions. Through knowledge and education (cognitive force domains), an individual can be transformed from a homeless to the CEO of an organization, from a college dropout to a software developer, and from a person with bigoted ideas to one with humanitarian dispositions.

What does radioactivity have to do with the cognitive force? It is not so much that a particle transmutes to another particle as it is the spark that is emitted in this reaction. It is the spark or radiation emitted that carries the energy and the message. Similarly in the human brain, one chemical is converted to another chemical; and in this transmutation, a biophoton is produced. Recent research, using newer technology such as biophoton modulation, is verifying earlier research on the works of biophotons.[1] It is showing that the thalamus and cerebral cortex do have neurons communicating among themselves with biophotons. These biophotons have a special name—*ultraweak photon emissions* (UPE).[2, 3] UPEs are produced by the decay of electrically excited neurons.[4] It so happens that the word *weak* in UPE and *weak* in the force of physics is a coincidence. This is not a case where neuroscience borrows from physics terminology.

Neurons have a body, dendrites (arms that receive messages), and axons (legs that send messages). Axons have a sheath with a high refractive index just like fiber-optic cables.[4] It is through these "fiber-optic cables" that the thalamus sends photons with bundles of information to the cerebral cortex, and vice versa. Thus, there is a large network of light-based communications between the thalamus and cerebral cortex, just as they are between the nucleus and electrons.

If you have doubts about lights traveling through your brain, close your eyelids and gently press on your eyeballs. Enact staring at the inside of your eyelids, and you will see flashes of light without even an external source of light. These light flashes are called *phosphenes*.[3, 5]

Just to clarify, we are using the thalamus and cerebral cortex as terminals for UPE transmission but all living biological systems (microbial, plant, and animal cells) emit UPE spontaneously.[6, 7] The human brain, however, can emit UPE spontaneously and induced. Spontaneous emission is when a crazy visual image pops up into the mind out of nowhere (e.g., visualize knocking the silly hat off Queen Elizabeth's head), or induced is when you deliberately visualize a plan of action (e.g., this weekend I envision myself sitting down in the kitchen table to study for my math test).

In the examples above, I have taken a quantum leap from UPE to visual images. Let me explain. Cognitive functions are a complex cooperative activity of many neurons that receive and send bundles of information.[2] Scientists have measured UPE using photometric instruments.[8] Studies are showing that UPEs correlate closely with electroencephalogram (EEG) waves, cerebral blood flow, cerebral metabolism, synaptic plasticity, neurotransmission, and memory formation.[3, 8–10] Prior to this technology, the source of EEG activity was obscure.[10] There is no other brain activity, like UPE, that has shown correlations with many cognitive functions.

An important role of UPE is the creation of visual images. We need to understand, however, that there are no real visual images in our minds. What we see and feel are sensations of visual images. These are only representations of reality or a subreality. Let me give you an example of subreality. Close your eyes and imagine seeing yourself standing on the beach, then walking barefoot on the sand, and looking at the ocean waves. You can even imagen these in color.

Where and how are visual images created? The brain weight is only 2 percent of the total body but uses 20 percent of the entire oxygen.[11] And within the brain the largest consumer of oxygen and energy are the synapses. Synapses are where most of the computing and memory storage occurs.[12] Once a presynaptic bouton fuses with the postsynaptic bouton to create a synaptic cleft, there is a burst of UPE emission in the synaptic cleft (the gap between pre- and post-synapses).[1, 13, 14] The work of several neuroscientists working in vision show that visual images are formed and sensed in the electrical field produced in the synaptic cleft. Synaptic clefts, like capacitors in an electrical circuit, produce an electronic field where energy is stored.

An analogy I can give in this regard is cathode rays and how these recreate images on a television.

The research on UPE is still evolving and much to be learned. But there are some indications that UPEs are associated with the production of REM dreams,[2] thinking,[8] meditation,[2, 7, 10] consciousness,[2, 7, 8] the bright light seen in near-death experiences[10] and, when UPE malfunction, involved with the visual hallucinations in schizophrenia.[2]

Communicative Force ≈ EM

EM force is the physical interaction that occurs between electrically charged particles. EM force is energy that travels through air and the vacuum of space. EM waves, like light and radiation, are made up of photons that carry discrete bundles of energy. Photons have no mass, travel at the speed of light, and are transmitters of messages. EM force can attract or repulse.

The communicative force, like EM, transfers energy in the form of messages from one individual or body to another. The communicative force consists of both language and nonlanguage communications. But it is through language that the communicative force transmits its strongest and clearest messages.

The processing center of the communicative force is the cerebral cortex. Language is a domain of the cerebral cortex. Talking and hearing are important parts of language, but it is through writing and reading that language is taken to an "atomic" level. The retina within the eye is an *electromagnetoreceptor*. Electromagnetoreceptors are hairs in the retina that detect photons. When a person is writing and reading, it is photons going back and forth between the paper and the retina passing bundles of information to the optic nerve from where it is relayed to the cerebral cortex via the thalamus. No need to say that language, like EM force, can be attractive or repulsive.

How the forces from the two sets (physics and human nature) recombined among themselves have some similarities too. At the beginning of the universe, the EM and weak force were combined into one (electroweak force). Similarly, the cognitive (thalamus) and communicative forces (cerebral cortex) are so interconnected that they can be seen as one unit. Later when the universe expanded into its current form, the strong force combined with the electroweak to form a superforce. Similarly, the affective (amygdala), cognitive (thalamus), and communicative (cerebral cortex) forces are all unified within the brain.

Socio-Environmental Force ≈ Gravity

Gravity is the curve in space-time caused by objects with mass. Because mass cannot be negative, the gravity from mass always attracts. The gravitational attraction of the original matter present in the universe caused it to coalesce to form stars and stars to form galaxies. Gravity is more closely related to the EM than to the strong and weak forces. The reason is that they both act on particles (masses or charges, respectively) and are carried by ripples of space.

The socio-environmental force emanates not from empty space but from all objects in the universe. The socio-environmental force tends to attract objects together into similar groups such as animal species and plant types; and among humans, they form clusters by race, culture, religion, politics, sports teams, and professional associations (just to name a few). People want to be attracted to one another and interact with other beings and nature.

The processing center of the socio-environmental force is the insula or insular cortex. Gravity affects the motion of all objects by accelerating them toward the center of the earth. Because gravity shapes our perception of where our body is relative to our environment, there needs to be a brain processing center to keep us in equilibrium.[15] That center is the insula. The insula is activated in tasks that involve gravity such as catching a fly ball, breaking a fall, feeling the acceleration of a speeding car, and going around a telephone post that is leaning. As I have stated throughout the book, all brain areas are interconnected. The cerebellum also plays an important role in reading the socio-environmental force, but it is the insula that is of the highest order.

The specialized nerve endings that capture the gravitational force are called *graviceptors* (or gravireceptors).[16, 17] Graviceptors are located primarily in the inner ear but are also found in joints, tendons, and muscles. The eyes also play a role in controlling body posture and movement. From these sensory organs, the gravitational force is sent up to the insula via the thalamus.[18] Just to reemphasize, the thalamus is supreme in cognition and depends on peer review—in this case, the insula—to stay in balance.

Like the link between gravity and EM, the socio-environmental force is more closely related to the communicative force than it is to the affective and cognitive forces. Similar to the communicative force, the socio-environmental force acts on objects and travels through the ripples of space.

As we have stated in the beginning and have stated in the end, science is an evolving field and what is true today might not be true tomorrow. And that brain sections are all interconnected. Although neurons from one brain section reach out to many other brain sections, in this book we attempted to simplify neuroscience by putting the spotlight on the predominant processing centers of each force.

Endnotes

1   Shainline, J. M. "Fluxonic processing of photonic synapse events." *IEEE Journal of Selected Topics in Quantum Electronics* 2020; 26 (1): 1–15.

2   Bókkon, I., Dai, J., and Antal, I. "Picture representation during REM dreams: a redox molecular hypothesis." *Biosystems* 2010; 100 (2): 79–86.

3   Wang, C., Bókkon, I., Dai, J., and Antal, I. "Spontaneous and visible light-induced ultraweak photon emission from rat eyes." *Brain Res.* 2011; 1369: 1–9.

4   Zarkeshian, P., Kumar, S., Tuszynski, J., Barclay, P., and Simon, C. "Are there optical communication channels in the brain?" *Front Biosci (Landmark Ed)* 2018; 23: 1407–1421.

5   Tang, R., and Dai, J. "Biophoton signal transmission and processing in the brain." *J Photochem Photobiol B.* 2014; 139: 71–75.

6   Cifra, M., and Pospíšil, P. "Ultra-weak photon emission from biological samples: definition, mechanisms, properties, detection and applications." *J Photochem Photobiol B.* 2014; 139: 2–10.

7   Sun, Y., Wang, C., and Dai, J. "Biophotons as neural communication signals demonstrated by in situ biophoton autography." *Photochem Photobiol Sci.* 2010; 9 (3): 315–322.

8   Dotta, B. T., Saroka, K. S., and Persinger, M. A. "Increased photon emission from the head while imagining light in the dark is correlated with changes in electroencephalographic power: support for Bókkon's biophoton hypothesis." *Neurosci Lett.* 2012; 513 (2): 151–154.

9   Rahnama, M., Tuszynski, J. A., Bókkon, I., Cifra, M., Sardar, P., and Salari, V. "Emission of mitochondrial biophotons and their effect on electrical activity of membrane via microtubules." *J Integr Neurosci.* 2011; 10 (1): 65–88.

10 Salari, V., Valian, H., Bassereh, H., Bókkon I., and Barkhordari A. "Ultraweak photon emission in the brain." *J Integr Neurosci.* 2015; 14 (3): 419–429.

11 Harris, J. J., Jolivet, R., and Attwell, D. "Synaptic energy use and supply." *Neuron* 2012; 75 (5): 762–777.

12 Cheng, Z., Ríos, C., Pernice, W. H. P., Wright, C. D., and Bhaskaran, H. On-chip photonic synapse. *Sci Adv.* 2017; 3 (9): e1700160.

13 Shainline, J. M., McCaughan, A. N., Buckley, S. M., Mirin, R. P., and Nam, S. W. "Superconducting optoelectronic neurons IV: transmitter circuits." *csNE* 2018; 2: 1–16.

[14] Miesenböck, G., and Rothman, J. E. "Patterns of synaptic activity in neural networks recorded by light emission from synaptolucins." *Proceedings of the National Academy of Sciences of the United States of America* 1997; 94 (7): 3402–3407.

[15] Teaford, M., Keller, K., and Merfeld, D. M. "The contribution of interoceptive signals to spatial orientation: A mini-review." *Neuroscience and Biobehavioral Reviews* 2022; 143: 104943.

[16] White, O., Gaveau, J., Bringoux, L., and Crevecoeur, F. "The gravitational imprint on sensorimotor planning and control." *J Neurophysiol.* 2020; 124 (1): 4–19.

[17] Cuturi, L. F. "Perceptual Biases as the Side Effect of a Multisensory Adaptive System: Insights from Verticality and Self-Motion Perception." *Vision (Basel)* 2022; 6 (3).

[18] Delle Monache, S., Indovina, I., Zago, M., Daprati, E., Lacquaniti, F., and Bosco, G. "Watching the Effects of Gravity. Vestibular Cortex and the Neural Representation of 'Visual' Gravity." *Front Integr Neurosci.* 2021; 15: 793634.

About the Author

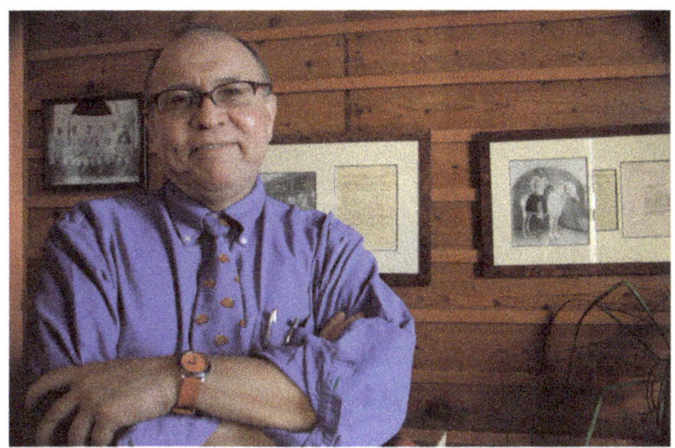

Roberto Treviño Peña, MD, received his medical degree from the Universidad Nacional Autónoma de México in Mexico City. He is residency-trained in internal medicine from the University of Health Sciences Center / Chicago Medical School and fellowship trained in critical care medicine from the Chicago Institute of Critical Care. In his critical care medicine training, his area of research was cardiopulmonary resuscitation and brain physiology.

After his specialty training, he returned to his hometown in San Antonio, Texas, where he founded the South Alamo Medical Group for the practice of medicine and the San Antonio Institute of Medicine to manage the business of the medical group. The medical group opened primary care clinics in the poorest neighborhoods of San Antonio. Despite increasing health care availability and newer medications, the incidence of chronic diseases such as diabetes and heart disease has continued to increase in all Americans but even more so among poor and minority populations. His research and that of others showed that 91 percent of causes of chronic disease were related to unhealthy behaviors. This led him to create the Social and Health Research Center Inc., a nonprofit center established to design and evaluate behavior modification programs to prevent chronic disease.

As for what gives him the expertise to touch on the subject of brain function and human behavior? He has been awarded $21 million of National Institutes of Health grants to conduct randomized trials aimed at modifying human behavior to prevent disease. Studies published from these trials have shown successful results in modifying unhealthy behaviors and risk factors for disease (www.sahrc.org). It is this experience and knowledge that Dr. Treviño Peña wants to share with the readers to help them live healthier, more productive, and saner life.